Rice and the Seven Day Rice Diet

by Lennie Richards, Al Bauman, Herman and Cornellia
Aihara, and Others

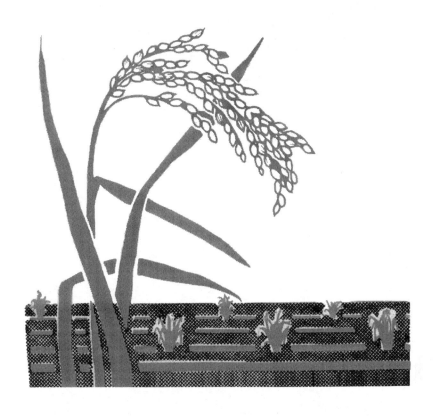

George Ohsawa Macrobiotic Foundation
Chico, California

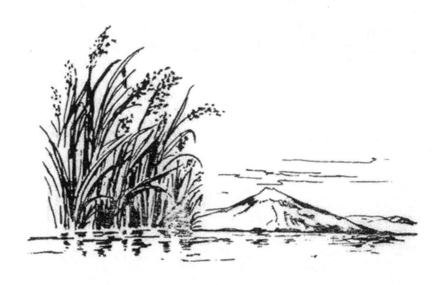

First Edition	1971
Second Printing	1975
Third Printing	1976
Current Edition, minor edits	2015 Jan 15

Published with the help of East West Center for Macrobiotics
   www.eastwestmacrobiotics.com

ISBN 978-0-918860-01-9

Printed in the United States of America

Contents

The Secret Of Macrobiotics

by George Ohsawa

People today praise the fantastic achievement of man's landing on the moon. We are all awed by the precision and accuracy of science and technology, and the courage of man that made this feat possible.

However, it seems to me, man himself is much more precise and fantastic. All of life is wonderful. The whole universe is much more precise in its movement and changes than any technology could be.

Man's heart pushes out four tons of blood over a distance from New York to Hong Kong every day, 365 days a year, throughout a whole lifetime without resting, heating up, or making noise.

Where and how does the heart get this energy?

Who built this fantastic heart, and how was it built?

Did you build your heart? If so, you must know how. If you don't know the way the heart is built, you must admit your ignorance. Awareness of this ignorance urges you to study and inspires a sense of wonder before nature. The awareness of the wonderfulness of nature and of man himself is the starting point of macrobiotics.

The tremendous power of the heart must come from the whole universe. The magical power that builds our heart must exist in our food. How does food do such a fantastic job? Nature performs this task quietly and precisely without any noise and without a billion dollar's worth of research.

Life is wonderful. Without food, there is no life. The right food gives a healthy and happy life.

This is the secret of macrobiotics.

Rice

by Lennie Richards

History Of Rice

Grains, the seeds of cereal plants, have been a staple food for man since time immemorial, and they are still the most important single class of foods throughout the world. The best known of these are rice, wheat, barley, oats, rye, corn, millet, and buckwheat.

Grains have been the main source of man's development, and their cultivation dates back before recorded history.

About seven or eight thousand years ago, in the early post-glacial period, gradual withdrawal of the arctic ice left fertile valleys and well-irrigated plains with a stable climate. The first areas freed of the arctic ice were in Southeast Asia; so while Europe and North America were still buried under tons of ice, the people of Southeast Asia were gathering grains for food. The prevailing climate was very suitable for the growth of cereal plants; and since the grains were small, dry, and compact, year-long storage was possible, insuring the populace of a continuous supply of food. So began the history of Man the agriculturist.

Because of its wonderful adaptability to different conditions, rice became the most popular grain and still ranks number one in cultivation, feeding more than one-third of the entire population of the world.

The earliest records of rice cultivation date back about 5,000 years to Ancient China. To these people, rice was more than daily food; it also played an essential role in their religious observances.

Rice cultivation in the Middle and Far East has always had a special meaning to the inhabitants of those areas. The Japanese deified it in the form of the ice-god Toyo-uke-no-okami. In some parts of India, it was used in ceremonial observances. Among Hindus, it was customary to make an offering of rice on the birth of a male child. The Javanese considered rice the offspring of their goddess

Dewi Sri, paying homage to her on many festive occasions. And the Sanskrit word for rice is dhanga—supporter or nourisher of Man.

From its beginnings in Eastern and Southern Asia, rice eventually spread throughout the entire world. India introduced it to Persia in about 400 B.C. The tradition of throwing rice at newlyweds originated in Persia. It was believed that this act insured happiness and prosperity. The Moorish invasion of Southern Europe brought rice to Spain; by 1470 it was being cultivated in Italy; Spain brought it to South America (Peru, Brazil, and the Guianas) in 1550; and it reached the shores of Virginia (then called 'English Colonial America') in 1694 and quickly spread to North and South Carolina, Georgia, Louisiana, and Texas. Rice was first planted in California in 1912, and has since become a major crop there.

Varieties

When we think of rice, we usually think of short-grain, long-grain, whole (brown), or polished (white). But there are actually thousands of varieties of rice. In Ceylon alone, there are 161 different varieties of rice. In China, India, and Japan, more than 1,400 exist. And since its introduction to this country about 250 years ago, several hundred different varieties have been cultivated.

Why so many different varieties of rice?

Different climates create different environmental conditions, which produce different soils—food for the growing rice plants. Short-grain rice, for example, naturally grows in colder climates, such as Belgium, Northern California, or Northern Japan, whereas long-grain grows more easily in warmer climates such as those of India, South China, or the Gulf States of America. Also, short-grain rice grows in high altitudes, while long-grain varieties grow in lowland and coastal areas.

Northern climates, high altitudes (yin) produce short-grain rice (yang).

Southern climates, lowlands and areas near the ocean (yang) produce long-grain rice (yin).

For an explanation of yin and yang, see *Macrobiotics: An Invitation to Health and Happiness* by George Ohsawa.

Structurally, all rice is basically the same, no matter what the variety. There are two major parts: the larger endosperm ('ko' in Japanese) and the smaller germ ('me' in Japanese). These two are then covered by seven layers of bran ('nuka'), which protect the grain and maintain its nutritional qualities by providing large amounts of proteins, fats, minerals, and vitamins.

Nutritional Content

Today, much rice, especially in Western countries, is cultivated with chemical fertilizers in order to produce a greater yield per acre. Western farmers are now producing more rice per acre than those who use more primitive methods.

The question is: just how beneficial is this? Which is more important—a higher yield per acre or a higher quality of rice?

Chemically-fertilized rice, though more abundant, is greatly inferior in quality. It lacks the strength and adaptive ability of rice grown without synthetic chemicals and thus is not able to adapt to and withstand storms, floods, and other climatic variables.

Also, through continued use of such chemicals, the plants are weakened, their transmutation/photosynthetic ability is very much reduced, and they consequently return far less minerals to the soil than under normal conditions. The soil is thus eventually depleted of minerals and is no longer able to sustain life. The farmer then puts more chemicals into the soil in order to build up the mineral content (especially nitrogen, essential in protein production) of the soil, thereby further acidifying it and making it more and more unproductive.

In the Orient, on the other hand, and especially in China and Japan until very recently, when unnatural agricultural techniques began becoming the rule, everything organic was put back into the soil: rice straw, weeds, manure—anything at all of organic origin available. And although the results of such natural agricultural techniques are lower yields and smaller grains, the nutritional content is much higher.

There have been many books written on rice and rice diets. They deal with cultivation, chemical breakdown, etc. These books certainly have merit and are well worth reading. But it should be kept in mind that the people who wrote them were not eating rice (especially brown [whole] rice) as their main food. Without the experience of eating rice as their daily food, these authors have dissected rice into its various components (proteins, carbohydrates, fats, minerals, vitamins, etc.), and have declared that it is lacking in certain factors:

> "Rice, like all other cereals, is not a complete food, even in the 'whole' unmilled state...it does not contain sufficient amounts of all the nutrients needed for health."
> – from *Rice and Rice Diets*, published by the Food and Agriculture Organization of the United Nations

This statement is certainly true of milled (white) rice, and is also true to an extent even of whole (brown) rice because: (1) Having greatly reduced his natural ability to produce (transmute) from whole rice the nutrients he needs to maintain a high degree of physical and mental health, the average person today does need at least small amounts of supplementary foods such as vegetables, beans, seaweeds, and even a little fish and fruit or nuts (about once or twice a week, depending on his condition, the weather, and other variables); (2) Even whole rice, if it has been grown with unnatural chemicals, as is most often the case today, is deficient in certain nutritional factors. There is a very big difference in nutritional value between rice that has been grown organically and that which has not; and (3) Other whole grains in combination with brown rice will definitely give a better balance of proteins, minerals etc. But it is also true that the nutritional value of whole rice has not been fully appreciated by modern Western nutritional science because nearly all commercially available rice has been subjected to milling processes whose purpose is to remove the outer branny layers, leaving little but the perishable starchy endosperm for human consumption. While it is not the purpose of this report to present statistics, it is true that the milling of brown rice in order to produce white rice (known as 'kasu,' waste of rice in Japanese) does remove very large amounts of certain essential nutrients so that a person who bases his diet on white rice definitely does need considerable amounts of supplementary foods; whereas, one whose principal food is brown rice will need much less additional foods. The following table shows the approximate percentages of important nutrients that are discarded in making brown rice into white rice:

Proteins 15%
Fats 85%
Calcium 90%
B Vitamins: niacin, pyridoxine, thiamine,
pantothenic acid, and riboflavin 55%-80%

For the past one hundred years or so, Orientals have abandoned their traditional brown rice for milled white rice.

Why did they change?

They must have forgotten why they were eating brown rice in the first place. Our freedom stems from understanding why we eat certain foods and avoid others. The Orientals had lost this understanding and were dominated by sensory judgment: a liking for the taste of white rice without regard for its value. Is it any wonder that, shortly after white rice came into fashion, beriberi and pellagra appeared? After intensive research by Western nutritionists, it was found that these diseases occur only when the body is deficient in B vitamins. Beriberi and pellagra were slowly eradicated with the introduction of unmilled and partially milled rice. On this point we are grateful for their extensive research.

On the other hand, modern Western nutritionists claim that even whole brown rice is incomplete.

How was this conclusion reached?

According to Western reasoning, the body must be adequately supplied with protein (Greek: protos—to come first). Since the human body is predominantly protein, which must be renewed every day, a good source is needed to maintain health. And it has been analytically 'proved' that since animal food contains a large quantity of such protein, a diet without animal food would be incomplete. What a strange mentality!

How do they account for the health of such herbivorous animals as elephants, cows, and horses who never eat animal food? Where do they get the protein to build such large bodies? Their diet of grasses alone contains very little protein (or calcium). But have you ever heard of an elephant suffering from protein or calcium deficiency?

To our understanding the answer is simple: their natural food is changed (transmuted) in their bodies into the nutrients they need to maintain their growth and health. (For more complete information concerning internal chemical change, please read *Biological Transmutation* by Louis Kervran.)

The following paragraphs, from *Vital Facts About Foods*, by Otto Carque, are in direct contradiction to current Western nutritional standards:

> While protein in its different forms is necessary for our nutrition, the required amount has been overestimated. The craving for concentrated protein foods like meat is one of man's acquired habits and has led to many diseased conditions.
>
> Since our muscular tissue consists mainly of protein, the early students of physiology supposed that this constituent was the source of muscular energy. In fact, it has been one the physiological dogmas of the past that tissues and organs of the body, or rather their constituent cells, must be supplied with protein for all their functions whenever possible.
>
> The remarkable fact that the output of nitrogen is equivalent to the intake of protein, and that the body cannot store up nitrogen to any considerable extent, has been mistaken as conclusive evidence that the organism prefers to use protein for most of its requirements.
>
> The painstaking investigations of Dr. M. Hindhede of Copenhagen, Denmark, published in his book, *Protein and Nutrition*, and of Dr. C. Roese, of Erfurt, Germany, *Over Consumption of Protein and Under Consumption of Basic Elements*, proved beyond doubt that normal body weight can be maintained and our health and endurance increased on an alkaline diet furnishing even less than

two ounces of protein per day. A diet high in protein and in other acid-forming foods means the consumption of heavy meals, an excess of waste products (which over-taxes the liver and kidneys), retarded elimination, and susceptibility to disease.

The low protein requirements of man's normal diet are also demonstrated by the changes which occur in moth-er's milk at the different stages of the infant's develop-ment. Under normal conditions, the mammary glands of the mother supply less protein as the infant grows older, so that after six months the percentage of protein in moth-er's milk has decreased from 2.4 to 1.1.

Furthermore, recent experiments in Japan, conducted by Dr. Kieichi Morishita (a physiologist specializing in the study of blood), indicate that carbohydrates change into protein and fat in our bodies and that an external supplement of animal protein is not necessary. (See *Hidden Truth of Cancer*, by K. Morishita, M.D.)

We should always remember that the principal food of Western man is meat and other animal food and that his mentality stems from his diet.

Why Do We Eat Rice?

As mentioned earlier in this article, the nutritional value of brown (whole) rice is far greater than that of milled (white) rice. We eat brown rice and other whole grains in order to establish and maintain our health. We use them as main foods in preference to animal foods because we want to establish peace within ourselves. Most grains (especially whole rice and wheat) contain a biochemical balance very similar to that of healthy human blood (in a temper-ate climatic zone). For example, the potassium/sodium ratio in both healthy human blood and in a diet mainly composed of whole grains and vegetables is about 10/1, (that of rice and wheat is about 7/1). By eating grains as our principal foods (about ½ of our diet), with vegetables as secondary foods (about ¼) and others (beans, sea veg-etables, fruits, nuts, fish, dairy products, and seasonings) filling out most of the remainder, our health and mental clarity improve and our supreme judgment (cosmic consciousness, awareness of Oneness) reveals itself. This is the natural state of Man: physical, mental, and spiritual health.

Those who base their diet on animal foods, on the other hand, tend to become involved in extremes of living and thinking, and to see only one side of a situation (the 'front'), rather than seeing both sides (the 'front' and the 'back'). To rely primarily on animal foods for building our body and brain cells (rather than transmuting those cells from mainly grains and other vegetable foods) makes us dependent and lazy—physically and mentally.

Some other disadvantages of animal products as main foods: the highly chemicalized foods most domesticated animals are now fed, the antibiotics with which they are injected, the hormones with which they are stimulated to grow quickly, the preservatives put in them after they are killed, and the extremely high costs of raising and processing them. Gradual conversion of land from animal food production to grain and vegetable production would be a very big step towards the establishment of peace on earth.

Storage

Harvested at the early stages of maturity, rice can be stored for one to five years without spoilage. It is recommended that about 3 grains out of 100 be green. The rice should then be allowed to dry until the moisture content is down to 12-14 percent. In storing rice for any length of time, it is advisable for it to remain with the husk on. It should be kept in a cool dry place, with good ventilation. In warm damp climates, rice should not be bought in too large a quantity, as it tends to become wormy.

Eastern Man And Western Man

Eating whole brown rice in order to re-establish one's health poses problems for the Western man not encountered by his Eastern counterpart, whose ancestors have been eating rice for thousands of years, and who has been following the Western way of eating for only a short time. It is thus much easier for an Oriental to return to his traditional food (grains) provided he wishes to do so.

Western man, on the other hand, has many generations of meat-eating within him, and the physiology of a meat-eater is quite different from that of a grain-eater. Meat is digested in the stomach and intestines, while grain is digested primarily in the mouth. It is necessary, therefore, for the former meat-eater to chew rice and other grains very thoroughly. Unchewed grains are extremely difficult to digest and assimilate; insufficient chewing leads to acidosis and other difficulties.

At the beginning of the change in diet, there may be signs of vitamin deficiency. This is not due to the incompleteness of the rice, but to the body's inability to produce the necessary elements. If this happens, eat a broader diet for a while: rice and other grains, vegetables, seaweed, beans, fish, and some nuts and fruit (preferably cooked), or even a little milk or cheese, if it is made from raw, whole milk and free of artificial chemicals. As your organism strengthens, it will eventually regain its ability to produce everything you need. As this happens, and as your backlog of meat (yang) diminishes, slowly but surely reduce the quantities and frequency of eating nuts, fruit, and dairy products, or you will become more and more yin. Also, try to keep fish to a minimum, as its consumption tends to limit our metaphysical (yin) thinking ability, and keep in mind that raw vegetables are much preferable to fruits, most of the time.

The Ten-Day Rice Diet
by Al Bauman

Although its effects may seem miraculous, the ten-day rice diet is not in the least mysterious.

The ten-day rice diet is not a fad; it is the first step on the road to changing one's life and dietary habits on a permanent basis. It is the door to an understanding of the Order of the Universe, the understanding of Macrobiotics.

The human body changes its blood stream every ten days. And in a relatively short period of time, the whole cellular structure of the body is renewed. It is thus possible to change the direction of your life in a few days. Instead of moving in a direct line from health to disease, you can reverse your field and progress from disease to health. Establish a sound blood stream and your path to well-being is assured.

In 1959, George Ohsawa visited the United States for the first time and gave lectures on macrobiotics. (The word refers to a large, over-all conception of life as opposed to a small, microscopic view.)

Mr. Ohsawa, concerned with both biological and philosophical questions, does not separate them. Together they express the unity of existence.

Whatever we do reflects our understanding of life—eating, drinking, thinking, working, praying. Mr. Ohsawa, recognizing the widespread need for practical application of a full understanding of life, proposes dietary changes as the concrete beginning point for action. Only a practical philosophy can lead to happiness and well-being in a continuously challenging life.

The principles that George Ohsawa has taught in his lectures and seminars throughout the world are based on Oriental philosophy five thousand years old, a tradition that sees all phenomena as the interplay of opposites...opposites that are the dynamics of life...opposites that are antagonistic and complementary.

The terms Yin and Yang, as used by Mr. Ohsawa, refer basically to the qualities of expansion and contraction. Within these two classifications are innumerably varied pairs of opposites: negative and positive, female and male, night and day, cold and hot, etc.

All phenomena can be classified according to Yin and Yang, including food and drink. They are made comprehensible and are seen as something more than what we take when we are hungry or thirsty. (Classification of foods is determined by color, shape, water content, climate of growth, direction and rate of growth, potassium-sodium content, etc.)

Health and happiness lie in the central area between extreme Yin and extreme Yang. The excitement of the center is that of the tightrope walker, but this central area is broader for us than the thin strand of wire that challenges the skill of the circus performer. Our understanding is constantly reshaped by the concept of balance and by the realization that our actions and judgment depend upon it.

Whole brown rice forms the core of the ten-day rice diet. Short grain is preferable. Rice hulled with rubber discs should be chosen over stone-hulled or steel-hulled rice, since it remains completely unscratched. Also, no talc (preservative) is used in packaging rubber-disced rice. See table on page 16.

For greatest health, happiness, and freedom, avoid extreme Yin and extreme Yang. These substances are very difficult for the body to neutralize. To avoid being attracted to very Yin substances, avoid very Yang substances. For good quality Yang, choose miso, tamari, and unrefined sea salt, used in moderation. For good quality Yin, choose salads, seeds, nuts, or temperate fruits occasionally. Foods from zone 2, slightly yin, are balanced by salt, heat, pressure, and time for the perfect balance, which is freedom.

Extreme Yang ▲▲▲	Very Yang ▲▲	Yang ▲	Balanced ☼	Yin ▶	Very Yin ▶▶	Extreme Yin ▶▶▶
refined salt	sea salt	poultry	whole grains	vegetables	natural beers	tropical fruits
	red meat	eggs		beans	dairy foods	dyed tea
	tamari	fish		seaweeds	fruit juice	soft drinks
	miso			bancha tea	vegetable oil	sugared foods
				seeds	coffee	sugar
				salads	spices	drugs
				nuts		preservatives
				non-tropical fruits		chemicals
						other alcohols
						hallucinogens
						(LSD and so on)

[See *Essential Guide to Macrobiotics* for a complete discussion on the Yin and Yang qualities of verious foods. – Ed.]

Grain Diet

by Herman Aihara

When George Ohsawa first visited this country in 1959, he brought a draft of a manuscript in English. I asked him what book it was. He said this was the English version of his famous *New Diet for Health and Happiness*, which had sold a million copies in Japan in about twenty years. He named this book *Zen Macrobiotics,* and he was looking for someone to correct and revise his English so that the writing would be understandable to Americans.

He asked the president of a vegetarian society in New Jersey to do the job but it didn't work out. He asked audiences who came to his seminars held in January, February, and March of 1960 in New York City. None would dare to do it. Finally, a lady who had high scholastic degrees from Oxford University in England, and who was also one of Ohsawa's devoted students, took the job. She typed the manuscript, which was then mimeographed and bound with the manual help of Mr. and Mrs. Ohsawa and myself. Thus the first 300 copies of *Zen Macrobiotics* came out.

In the chapter called "10 ways of good Eating and Drinking," he states, "There are 10 ways of eating and drinking by which you can establish a healthy and happy life, if you know how to establish a good equilibrium of yin-yang in accordance with our philosophy of the orient. But even without understanding the theory, you can choose any of these 10 ways of "Health to Happiness" by observing these macrobiotic directions very carefully."

The 10 ways of good Eating and Drinking are shown in the chart on page 18.

If one looks at this chart carefully, one will realize that these 10 ways of diet include the diets of many countries. Because Ohsawa recommended the highest number as the easiest, simplest, and wisest, #7 diet became one of the most famous diets in America. Those who read *Zen Macrobiotics* tried to follow #7 diet but not so much

Ten Ways to Health and Happiness

diet #	cereals	vegetable nitsuke	soup	animal	salads fruits	dessert	drinks
7	100%						minimal
6	90%	10%					
5	80%	20%					
4	70%	20%	10%				
3	60%	30%	10%				
2	50%	30%	10%	10%			
1	40%	30%	10%	20%			
-1	30%	30%	10%	20%	10%		
-2	20%	30%	10%	25%	10%	5%	
-3	10%	30%	10%	30%	15%	5%	

the other lower diets. Unfortunately, several people's conditions got worse by strictly observing #7 diet (according to their doctor's reports). The worst thing happened when one young girl died after following #7 diet rigidly. Although she had been taking many drugs and observed fasting between #7 diet, the macrobiotic diet was solely blamed by her parents and doctors.

After this happened, macrobiotic leaders in this country started to warn people not to start #7 diet when they were new to Macrobiotics. It seems to me this change made Macrobiotics safer but less effective. #7 diet really works. Rather, it works too much.

Why Did Ohsawa Recommend #7 Diet?

I asked him why he recommended #7 diet one day at my New York home where he had been staying. He answered me simply, "It is the safest way of diet." He had experienced that #7 diet was safest in Europe.

I know Ohsawa was a very practical man. He never gave advice out of his head. His advice always came out of his many experiences and observations. He must have experienced that #7 diet was safest. We learned #7 diet was not safest in America. Why?

In my opinion, physiological conditions of Americans were worse than those of Europeans (whom Ohsawa taught before com-ing to America) because of deterioration of foods, pollution of water and air, disorderliness of living, and increasing drug use.

Americans, as well as Europeans, have been eating meat, dairy products, and white bread for many years. Thus, their biological constitution and their physiological functions are adapted to such foods. When they completely change to an Oriental diet—namely Macrobiotics—their digestive systems may not function well. Many orientals lived solely on rice and a few vegetables for many years. Rice is a highly nutritious food. It has proven to be so in the Orient. However, the #7 diet (grain and a little liquid) is perhaps the same as fasting for many modern people, especially Americans, because in the beginning they cannot assimilate its food value completely.

(Fasting is a good remedy for many sicknesses, as stated in *Fasting Cure* by Upton Sinclair. However, fasting can sometimes cause very strong and drastic changes for modern Americans, especially those who have damaged their nervous system by long usage of drugs.)

Since rice alone lacks the quantity of protein or essential amino acids we need for maintaining the body, it activates the body cells and organs to look elsewhere. The body uses up any usable items we have in our body. Waste products or excess storage are dug out to use. As the result, #7 diet often throws wastes or toxins into the blood stream. This is a good thing over short periods of time. However, should the kidneys and liver be weak, those wastes and toxins will circulate in the blood instead of being eliminated from the body and cause various ill effects. Loss of energy and tiredness commonly happen. If those toxins go to the throat, there will be coughing. One may feel depressed if these toxins go to the brain.

Not only the kidneys and liver are affected. Most Americans today are too weak or sensitive in their nerve center—the interbrain, which receives stimulation and sends out controlling messages to all organs. This is more so when they have taken marijuana or LSD.

The interbrain influences the pituitary gland, and the pituitary gland controls the adrenal gland of which the cortex controls Na^+, Cl, K^+ absorption in the kidney, and carbohydrate, protein, and fat metabolism. Should the interbrain be weak or too sensitive, it sends out stimulation to the pituitary gland in a much exaggerated manner.

The final result is lack of control of Na^+, Cl, K^+ absorption and un-balanced metabolism of carbohydrate, protein, and fat.

For example, a small decrease of glucose in the blood (this is a yang condition) will cause a strong stimulation of the adrenal gland, which will produce much cortical hormone (this is a yin condition) and change glycogen to glucose, causing the glucose level of the blood to become very high (this is a yin condition—the heart beat becomes faster, blood pressure rises). Yang → Yin

Then the high glucose (yin) level in turn stimulates the pancreas to produce insulin (yang) from the islets of Langerhans.

This insulin changes glucose to glycogen and stores it in the liver, or insulin helps glucose to enter cells. As the result, the glucose level again goes down (yang). Yin → Yang

Consequently, one swings from yin to yang and yang to yin incessantly. The more sensitive (yin) interbrain one has, the more faster, larger (yin) swinging he will get. He is emotionally unstable and nervous. For such a person, #7 diet is probably too yang a diet. Therefore, he is attracted to strong yin foods or liquid such as sugar or beer; and after eating or drinking such strong yin, he is depressed with a guilty feeling. The yin condition attracts strong yang such as meat or salty foods. He swings back and forth not only physiologically but also psychologically. Such cases Ohsawa had not expected.

The most dangerous effect of #7 diet, however, is when the diet is combined with fanatic persons. #7 diet has some effect to cause exclusive or a solitary attitude. One boy I know of stopped all social activities and stayed at home without going out for 3 years. In his case he was not strictly on #7 diet. Some will not listen to another's advice. He continued the diet against others' advice to stop, rigidly believing he was right. This attitude is not caused by #7 diet solely, but #7 diet seems to me to bring out such nature and makes it more apparent when he has it. In our past experiences, only such a case caused dangerous trouble. One who has fanatic and exclusive tendencies, therefore, should not follow #7 diet at all.

Benefit of #7 Diet

Although a few have had trouble with #7 diet, most who tried #7 diet received tremendous benefits. The following are some of the benefits they got. However, as stated before, some people may not get such good results.

1. Reduction of excess weight. Almost all over-weight people reduced their weight to a normal weight, even though many of them did not follow strictly #7 diet.

2. Almost all people experienced a better feeling, a clear mind, and detachment from worries.

3. Many felt energetic and found it easy to walk and run.

4. It cures constipation. People are constipated when they eat refined foods because there is no roughage to stimulate bowel movement in the large intestine. Whole grains, especially rice, have much roughage, which causes the movement.

Sugar vs. Grain Diet

#7 diet will balance out sugar (or glucose) metabolism. Glucose metabolism is controlled by two hormones, namely insulin and cortical hormone. Insulin is secreted from the pancreas and transfers blood glucose into the body cell. Therefore, it decreases blood glucose. Cortical hormone is secreted by the adrenal gland and increases glucose of the blood by changing glycogen to glucose. By these two hormones, blood maintains a constant glucose level—100 mg/100 cc (percent).

The increase of glucose in the blood causes an increase of insulin, which in turn causes above mentioned reactions and ends up with decreased glucose. This condition stimulates the adrenal gland to produce cortical hormone, which increases glucose in the blood by changing glycogen into glucose. When sugary foods are eaten, glucose in the blood increases very rapidly. As the result, much insulin is secreted from islets of Langerhans, and glucose enters the cells to lower blood glucose. This is hypoglycemia. In other words, too much sugar may cause low sugar in the blood. Such a person feels depressed after a short energetic active feeling.

On the other hand, grains turn to glucose slowly in the digestive canal and increase blood glucose slowly. Therefore, no great amount of insulin is secreted, and no low level of glucose in the blood occurs. In other words, the glucose level stays fairly constant in the case of grain eating.

A grain diet brings a fairly constant condition of the metabolic state and mental mood. One is rarely upset even in emergency cases because blood sugar level tends to stay constant.

Also, sugar contains no minerals. Therefore, when sugar is eaten, the body's stored minerals must be drawn into the blood to maintain blood alkaline. In other words, sugar robs the body of minerals, especially calcium. Whole grains (not refined) contain such minerals. Therefore, although they are acid-forming foods, they will alkalize easily.

Grain vs. Acid and Alkaline

Grains are acid-forming foods. Therefore, a grain diet requires some alkaline-forming foods. Alkaline-forming foods are fruits, vegetables, seaweeds, seeds, miso, tamari, salt. Therefore, George Ohsawa recommended sesame salt with grains, so that the alkaline forming sesame salt would alkalize the body fluid. When making a balance of alkaline-forming foods and acid-forming foods, one must consider also the yin-yang of foods.

Yin alkaline-forming foods should balance with yang acid-forming foods—for example—fruits with meat. Yang alkaline-forming foods should balance with yin acid-forming foods. For example, miso, tamari, or salt with grains. (Note: grains are yin when compared with salt, miso, or tamari. However, they are yang when compared with vegetables).

Most Americans eat much acid-forming foods at dinner, such as meat, chicken, cheese, and they have difficulty waking up in the morning (acidic condition). Then they have to drink coffee or fruit juice at morning to wake up. (These are strong alkaline-forming foods.) By observing the diet given in this book, one will not need to drink coffee in the morning, and an alkaline condition will be maintained easily.

Grain and Protein

Grains are one of the most important sources of protein in the East. They contain a fairly good amount of protein, and the proportion of Essential Amino Acids (EAA) is good in most grains.

However, in order to reach the Minimum Daily Requirement

(MDR) of EAA, one has to eat about one pound of grains per day, which is too much for most Westerners. Therefore, #7 diet will cause a shortage of EAA in the long run. Many feel a craving for some animal foods after a certain period of #7 diet. This craving is a sign of lack of EAA. Therefore, it is better to satisfy the craving by eating a little amount of what is craved. Usually this craving will disappear by eating small amounts of such foods.

There are many delicious recipes using only grains or grains with a few vegetables. Observing such a diet will rejuvenate the body. Since it may cause cravings for some animal foods, I have added some animal foods for the beginners of a macrobiotic diet. In the recipes beginning on page 30, I calculated the amount of methionine and cystine, which are the lowest amount of EAA contained mostly in grains and other foods. The percentage of methionine and cystine in foods compared with MDR of EAA (methionine and cystine) determines what percentage of your protein is usable. [Current thinking is that lysine is the limiting EAA for grains. We have left the original calculations using methionine and cystine because foods high in these EAAs are also high in lysine. –ed.]

In the recipes beginning on page 30, I calculated such percentages. By these figures, you can see the percentage of MDR in each meal. If you are getting too low a percentage in meals, you should add some protein-rich foods such as miso, soy sauce, natto, wheat gluten, etc. The MDRs recommended by the National Research Council of the National Academy of Science, Washington, D.C. ("Evaluation of Protein Nutrition, Publication 711") are as follows:

Tryptophan	.250 grams
Threonine	.500 grams
Isoleucine	.700 grams
Leucine	1.100 grams
Lysine	.800 grams
Methionine	.200 grams
Methionine + Cystine	1.100 grams
Phenylalanine	.300 grams
Phenylalanine + Tyrosine	1.100 grams
Valine	.800 grams

For further information, read *Miso and Soy Sauce for Flavor and Protein* by Herman and Cornellia Aihara, published by the George Ohsawa Macrobiotic Foundation. This book contains recipes for making protein-rich foods listed before (miso, soy sauce, natto, wheat gluten, and so on.)

The values of Essential Amino Acids in the following evaluation of MDR% are based on *Protein and Amino Acid Content of Foods*, published by the Department of Agriculture, and *Food Values of Portions Commonly Used* by Bowes and Church, published by J. B. Lippincott. Co., and *Amino Acid Content in Japanese Food*, published by the Japanese Scientific Research Council.

Home Grown Rice

by Junsei Yamazaki and David Spiekerman

Growing rice in Chico, California this summer was exciting and surprisingly simple. Inspired by the giant rice paddies of Northern California, Junsei and I decided to plant a small 10' by 20' paddy of short-grain rice by traditional Japanese methods. We used no chemicals, poisons, or machines to grow our rice. By preparing the seed and rice paddy carefully and then giving our loving attention to the watering of the growing plants, we created a bountiful harvest of many delights. Standing before the dark green rice plants often warmed our hearts and affirmed the intimate friendship between rice and man. We are grateful to the countless farmers before us who created the green power and beauty of rice and who enabled us to experience the miracle of 'one grain, ten thousand grains'.

We prepared our rice seed in late March by a unique process. Taking about two pounds of seed Junsei had brought from Japan years ago, we separated the strong seed from the weak thusly: placing the seed in a bucket, adding cool water to the top, adding a few tablespoons of sea salt, and then swirling with our hands the entire mixture for a minute, we made the yang seed fall to the bottom and the yin seed float to the top of the bucket. We threw off the yin seed and swirled until no more seed floated on the water. Then we washed the salt away from the rice with cool water and a wire-strainer.

Next, we soaked the seed outdoors for three weeks. Placing the yang seed in a small cloth bag and tying it closed with string, we put the bag in a bucket with a three pound stone on top of it. Filling the bucket to the brim with water, we kept a tiny flow of water entering and circulating through the bucket by placing a hose in the bucket. Rice does not like stagnant water. The temperature of the water was always cool. We checked the bucket daily to insure the slight flow of water.

By the third week in April, we removed the seed from the soaking water. Opening the bag, we saw tiny, white sprouts at one end of every seed. For one day, we let the seed rest outside in the sun and air, drying a little. The germinating condition of the rice suggested the strength of the seed that had started to grow in cool water for three weeks. What other seeds can grow in such conditions for so long?

The next day, we planted the seed in a seedling bed. We chose a sunny, warm bit of soil 2' by 4'. With a simple hoe, we removed about 3 inches of the top layer of soil. We added leaf mold, animal manure compost, sand, and water to the bed. The compost was full of succulent earth worms. Then we scattered the seed by hand evenly over the bed. On top of the seed, we scattered sand thinly. Over the sand, we neatly placed rice straw and fastened it securely with a string to the ground to prevent the wind from blowing the seed away. Around the entire bed we posted a white string to spook any birds wishing to feast on the tiny green shoots soon to emerge.

The seedling bed received some rainfall, but we augmented it with regular watering every two days. By one week, the tender shoots broke through the sand. After 35 days, the plants were 4 to 5 inches tall. We were ready to transplant the green beauties to our paddy.

We located our paddy on ground that had been under lawn grass for countless years. It was clean and fertile soil. The paddy was 4' from our well, which had an unlimited supply of cold water. The drawbacks to the location were two: the paddy was situated on the north, shady side of large, leafy almond trees and did not receive full, direct sunlight until afternoon; and there was no space to warm the cold well water in a warming basin before it entered the paddy. Ideally, the water should be warm to promote the vigor and health of the growing rice.

One day before transplanting, we began preparing the soil and building the dikes for the paddy. With a spade, we worked the soil to a loose, friable condition. Then we dug a trench, 1.5' deep and six inches wide, along the perimeter of the paddy. The soil removed from the trenches became the dikes that we built along the outer side of the trenches. Then we put sheets of plastic down in the trenches against the outer walls of the trenches to retard seepage from the paddy to the bone dry ground outside. Into the trenches, next, we pushed the soil that remained between the trenches. See diagram (side view):

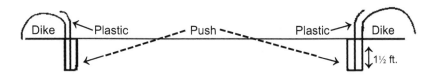

Thus, the paddy bottom was lower than the ground level and about ten inches lower than the tops of the dikes. We smoothed the paddy bottom level with a flat board and established the even flatness of the bottom with a trial flooding to determine the way the water acted.

The afternoon of May 26 was hot when we transplanted the seedlings. Removing the seedlings from the soil by hand, being careful not to damage their roots, we carried them to the paddy. We flooded the paddy to get the soil muddy. Marking off 14 rows eight inches apart in the paddy, three of us moved down the rows, plunging clumps of two or three plants into the mud six inches apart. This stoop labor took 20 minutes to complete. We actually planted about 1550 seedlings, which originated from three ounces of rice seed. Of those plants in the seedling bed, we transplanted 113 of them into the rice paddy. The rice was happy to be in the mud.

The plants spent a week establishing their roots firmly in the mud. Sometimes a plant would lose its hold and float on the water, but we simply placed it standing again, and it thrived. We flooded the paddy to a depth of one inch. Our technique used conservative amounts of water. We kept a moderate flow of water running into the paddy all day long because the water percolated slowly through the soil. It took us about one hour to fill the paddy in the morning with the tap turned to full. We turned the water off in the evening.

After 20 days of all day flooding, we cut the watering to half a day in the morning for another 20 days. Our purpose was to permit the afternoon sun to warm the soil around the base of the rice plants. The sun's warmth, without the layer of cool water, stimulated the growth of new plants. Each seed was capable of producing 12 more plants under the right conditions. We planted two to three plants per clump; by mid-July, each-clump was showing 10 to 20 new plants. The fecundity of this rice was amazing to behold.

The rice grew about two feet from mid-June to early August. Compared to chemical rice, our rice grew at an even pace. Commercial growers flood their paddies six inches or more. They use a formidable arsenal of herbicides, pesticides, fungicides, and chemical fertilizers to maintain the life of their paddies. These poisons were never needed in our rice paddy. Once a gopher broke through the paddy, and it took a few moth balls and buckets of soil down his hole to discourage his return. Then a Great Dane ate a foot off the tops of 30 plants on his stroll through the paddy, but the strength of these injured darlings replaced the lost foliage in a week's time to be equal with the height of the uninjured rice. Frogs, grasshoppers, butterflies, and myriad other insects made the paddy their home. Our cats slept in the cool paddy in the hot afternoons. We weeded only twice. Regulating the water level was our primary role as farmers. The rice took care of itself.

In early August, the first heads of grain appeared at the sunnier, northern end of the paddy. The flowering and self-pollination of the plants was not retarded by excessive rains or winds. When near-gale winds blew across Chico a few times during the summer, our rice stood tall, never breaking or permanently bending. About 5% of the new seeds were barren or insect damaged. By early September, all of the rice had headed. The heads started to turn yellow by mid-September and the heavy maturing panicles of grain bent downward. We stopped flooding the paddy on September 21 and allowed the paddy and rice to dry for one month longer than necessary.

On October 19, we harvested the rice using sickles and bundled it by hand. It took us one hour. We built a thresher out of wood and a metal grate. Beating a bundle of rice a dozen times against the grate, we finished threshing in one hour. We cleaned the rice by placing it on a plastic sheet, lifting it, and throwing it up in the windy air. For one week, the rice dried outside in the sun.

Chico's climate allowed us to keep the rice in the ground a long time. Supposedly, a minimum of 40 days with temperatures of 70 degrees Fahrenheit or more is required to grow short-grain rice. Our paddy was 1/215 of an acre, so one acre of rice grown using our method will yield 6450 pounds per acre if you plant 40 pounds of seed. The commercial, organic rice growers get 2500 pounds per acre, planting 100 to 200 pounds per acre by airplane. The chemical rice growers get 6000 pounds per acre. By any test, our method was economical and productive. We recommend growing rice to anybody who likes gardening. The remarkable power of rice will unfold before your eyes.

Recipes

by Cornellia Aihara

---

1. How to Cook a Small Amount of Rice in a Pressure Cooker

> 2 cups rice
> 3 cups water
> ½ tsp salt

After washing rice, soak in 3 cups of water for 1 hour in a 6-inch diameter stainless steel mixing bowl or any kind of pan that will fit in a 4 quart pressure cooker. Add the salt, then put 2 cups of water into a 4 quart pressure cooker. Place the mixing bowl in the pressure cooker. Lock the cover on, and bring to a boil over high flame. After 3 minutes, when pressure comes up to full, continue cooking over high flame for 15 minutes. Then cook 20 minutes more over a medium flame. Shut off flame, set for 20 minutes, take off the cover, and serve. This rice is not so sticky—good for summer.

Food	Amount	Protein	Methionine/Cystine gm.
Brown rice	2 cups	29.6	0.94
MDR%			85%

---

2. Pressure Cooked Rice (Serves 3)

> 1 cup brown rice
> 1 to 1½ cups water
> ¼ tsp salt

Rinse the rice as above. If your pressure cooker does not have much pressure, it is best to soak the rice overnight. Add the salt just before cooking. Cook on a low heat for 30 minutes. Then turn to high until pressure comes up to full. Lower heat and cook 45-60 minutes. Then turn off heat and allow pressure to return to normal, 20-30 minutes.

Remove cover and mix rice thoroughly before serving. (When cooking more than 10 cups of rice, decrease amount of water.)

Food	Amount	Protein	Methionine/Cystine gm.
Brown rice	1 cup	14.8	0.47
One serving		4.9	0.16
MDR%			14%

3a. Baked Rice (Serves 5)

> 2 cups brown rice
> 4 cups boiling water
> ½ tsp salt

Preheat oven to 350 degrees. Wash the rice, then dry roast in a heavy skillet over a medium flame until golden colored. Place the rice in a casserole and add salt and cover with boiling water. Cover pan and set in oven. Bake for one hour. This preparation is very soft and light and a pleasant change from pressure cooked rice. Because the rice comes out so light and fluffy, it prevents overeating.

Food	Amount	Protein	Methionine/Cystine gm.
Brown rice	2 cups	29.6	0.94
One serving		5.9	0.19
MDR%			17%

3b. Variation (Serves 5)

> 2 cups brown rice
> ¼ cup dried green peas
> 5 cups water
> 1 tsp salt

Wash peas and soak overnight or for about 5-6 hours in one cup of water. Wash and dry roast the rice and place in a casserole. Boil the remaining water with the salt and pour over rice. Cover casserole and place in a preheated 350 degree oven and bake for one hour.

If using fresh green peas, cook rice as above in regular baked rice recipe and add 1 cup fresh green peas, 2 tsp soy sauce, and ¼ tsp extra salt during the last 10 minutes of cooking.

Food	Amount	Protein	Methionine/Cystine gm.
Brown rice	2 cups	29.6	0.94
Green peas	¼ cup	7.6	0.14
Total		37.2	1.08
One serving		7.4	0.21
MDR%			19%

---

4. Boiled Brown Rice (Serves 7)

> 4 cups brown rice
> 6 cups water
> 1 tsp salt

Ideally, a porcelain coated cast iron, or heavy cast iron pot is best, although a stainless steel pan can also be used.

Rinse the rice gently in a pan of cold water, keep changing the water and rinsing until the water is clear. Soak rice overnight in the 6 cups of water. Add salt just before cooking. Cook on low heat for 30 minutes, then turn heat to high until boiling point is reached. Now cook for 20 minutes on a medium high heat and 40 minutes on low heat. Turn off heat again and let sit for 20 minutes. Remove cover and mix rice thoroughly before serving.

Food	Amount	Protein	Methionine/Cystine gm.
Brown rice	4 cups	59.2	1.88
One serving		8.4	0.269
MDR%			24%

Rice Cream

Prepared rice cream flour can be purchased in natural food stores, and at macrobiotic outlets, but it is very easy to prepare at home and tastes much fresher. To make the flour, wash the rice and dry roast in a heavy skillet (without oil) until it is golden colored and begins to pop. Either grind in an electric blender set at high speed or else grind by hand in a grain mill.

---

5. Rice Cream Cereal (Serves 4)

> 1 cup rice cream flour
> 3½ to 4 cups boiling water
> ¼ tsp salt

Dry roast the flour in a heavy skillet over a medium flame until it gives off a nut-like fragrance. Bring the pan to the sink. Add boiling water and salt. Mix quickly to remove lumps and return pan to heat. Cook over a low heat with a cover for 40-50 minutes, stirring occasionally to prevent burning. Mix thoroughly before serving.

Food	Amount	Protein	Methionine/Cystine gm.
Rice cream	1 cup	14.8	0.47
One serving		3.7	0.12
MDR%			10%

---

6. Thick Rice Cream (Serves 3)

> 1 cup rice cream flour
> 2 cups boiling water
> ¼ tsp salt

Roast the flour as above. Bring pan to sink to cool, then add salt and one cup boiling water. Mix quickly to prevent lumping. Return pan to heat and push aside the dough mixture with a rice paddle and add second cup of boiling water so that the dough floats above the water, and avoids contact with the bottom of the pan. Cover with a closely fitting lid and let rice steam over a low heat for 30-45 minutes. Mix thoroughly before serving.

Food	Amount	Protein	Methionine/Cystine gm.
Rice cream	1 cup	14.8	0.47
One serving		4.9	0.16
MDR%			14%

7. Rice Cream Cereal Variation

> 1 cup rice cream flour
> ½ cup sweet brown rice cream flour
> 4 to 4½ cups boiling water
> ⅓ to ½ tsp salt

This rice cream flour is not available to be purchased. The recipe was created by Cornellia Aihara and served at breakfast at G.O.M.F. Prepare the brown rice per instructions in the introductory paragraph to Rice Cream recipes. Wash the sweet brown rice and dry roast it separately from the brown rice, as the sweet brown rice requires less time to roast. Combine with the roasted brown rice in proportions of two pans brown rice to one pan sweet brown rice. Cook as in recipe #5 after grinding into rice cream flour.

Food	Amount	Protein	Methionine/Cystine gm.
Rice cream	1 cup	14.8	0.47
Sweet brown rice cream	½ cup	7.4	0.23
Total		22.2	0.70
One serving		5.5	0.14
MDR%			12%

8. Parsnip Rice Cream Casserole

Cook rice cream per usual. Slice parsnips on the diagonal and sauté until tender. In a casserole, place a layer of rice cream, next put a layer of sautéed parsnips that have been seasoned with salt and/or tamari, add another layer of rice cream, a second layer of parsnips. Sprinkle bread crumbs on top; place in a preheated 350 degree oven and bake 20-30 minutes until golden brown on top.

Rice Balls

Rice balls are good for picnics and traveling. Cold rice usually doesn't taste good but becomes tasty when made into rice balls. Sometimes it is difficult for pregnant women to eat rice, but they can usually eat it in the form of rice balls because a rice ball compresses the rice and makes it more yang. They become filled with the ki, or life energy, of the person making them.

George Ohsawa used to cure sick people by serving them rice balls. One rice ball was cut into 10 pieces and each piece was chewed 100 to 200 times. This helped sick people recover quickly. When you try to cure sick people, however, you must feel a deep, sincere desire that the sick person get better because this feeling is transmitted to the rice.

9. How to Make Rice Balls

Hot rice is best for rice balls. Fill a small rice bowl with rice; this is a good way to measure the correct amount to use. Don't squeeze rice balls too hard when you shape them. Use your shoulder muscles instead of squeezing with your fingers. Your fingers should just shape the rice. The rice should be firm on the outside and soft in the center.

Before making rice balls, your hands should be clean. If you wash with soap, make sure you completely rinse your hands to avoid soapy-tasting rice balls. Put bancha tea in a bowl, wet your hands in the tea, and hold the rice in your left hand. In the center, put two to three pieces of tamari kombu or a piece of salt plum for flavor. The salt plum keeps the rice from spoiling.

Cut nori into nine pieces and cover rice balls with toasted nori, gomashio, and pickled shiso leaves.

Use two pieces for one rice ball. Don't wet your hands too much with tea or the rice will get soggy and spoil easily.

See illustration on the page 36.

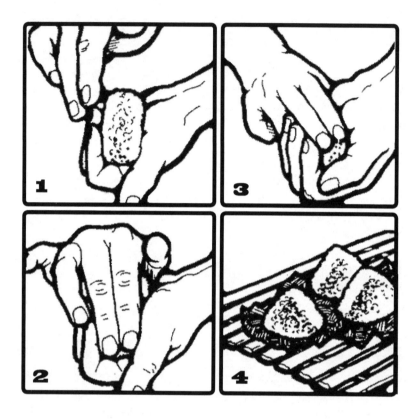

10. Azuki Bean Rice (Serves 5)

> 1⅔ cups rice
> ⅓ cup azuki beans
> ¼ to ½ tsp salt
> 3 cups water

Wash azuki beans and rice until water drains clear. Soak for 2 hours in 3 cups water before cooking, then cook as in recipe #1. Many people say that 2 cups of regular rice does not cook well in a 4 quart pressure cooker, but this combination comes out really well. This is a good way to cook a small amount of rice.

Food	Amount	Protein	Methionine/Cystine gm.
Brown rice	1⅔ cups	25.90	0.82
Azuki beans	⅓ cup	2.00	0.04
Total		27.90	0.86
One serving		5.5	0.17
MDR%			15%

11. Chestnut Rice (Serves 7)

    5 cups brown rice
    7 cups water
    1 lb fresh chestnuts
    2½ tsp salt
    8" strip of dashi-kombu, cut partway through every one
        inch like this:

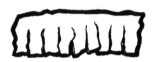

Soak unhulled chestnuts overnight and take off the dark outer skin and inside papery skin. If they are large, cut them in half.

In a pressure cooker, bring 7 cups of water and kombu to a boil. Remove kombu, add washed rice, salt, and gently stir well. Then put the cover on and cook for 20 minutes on a low flame. Then turn the flame up high until pressure comes up. After pressure is up, turn the flame down low and cook for 45 minutes. Shut off flame and, when pressure comes down, remove the cover and serve immediately.

Food	Amount	Protein	Methionine/Cystine gm.
Brown rice	5 cups	74.0	2.35
Chestnuts		Not available	Not available
One serving		10.5	0.33
MDR%			30%

12. Walnut Rice (Serves 10)

> 5 cups brown rice
> 1½ cups walnuts
> ⅓ cup soy sauce

Grind walnuts in a suribachi until half ground, add soy sauce, and grind again for about 10 minutes until they are just a little lumpy.

After rice is cooked, take off cover and spread walnut sauce on top. Replace cover and set for 5 minutes. Then mix rice and walnut sauce and serve. The combination is good with green vegetable ohitashi, clear soup, any kind of pickles (Takuan or miso), or toasted nori.

Food	Amount	Protein	Methionine/Cystine gm.
Brown rice	5 cups	74.0	2.35
Walnuts	1½ cups	22.5	0.46
Soy sauce	⅓ cup	5.2	0.10
Total		101.7	2.91
One serving		10.2	0.29
MDR%			26%

13. Bancha Rice—Pressure Cooked (Serves 7)

> 7 cups strong bancha tea
> 1⅓ tsp salt
> 5 cups brown rice

After washing rice, mix with bancha tea, and cook the same as for chestnut rice. If you don't have a pressure cooker, you must add 1 or 2 more cups of water. (See recipe #4.)

Food	Amount	Protein	Methionine/Cystine gm.
Brown rice	5 cups	74.0	2.35
One serving		10.6	0.34
MDR%			30%

14. Ohagi (Serves 5)

> 3 cups sweet brown rice
> ½ cup white sesame seeds
> 3 cups water
> 3 sheets of nori
> 1 tsp salt
> 1 Tbsp tamari
> 1 cup azuki beans
> 5 Tbsp Yinnie syrup

Wash azuki beans; place in a pan with 1½ cups water to soak overnight. Bring the beans to a boil in the pot, then add ½ cup of water. Bring to another boil. Add another ½ cup of water; bring to boil (three times in all). Then cook for 1 hour in a covered pot. Azuki beans are yang, so it is better to cook them in a pot than in a pressure cooker. Cooked in a pressure cooker, they become bitter. After 1 hour, add the Yinnie syrup to the azuki beans, uncover, and cook for 20 minutes, add ½ tsp salt, and cook for 5-10 minutes more. If you don't want a sweet taste, add salt only. Wash the sesame seeds and strain them. Put a sponge under the strainer to absorb the excess water. Roast the sesame seeds in a dry pan until they stop popping. Put them in a suribachi, add soy sauce, and grind until about half the seeds are ground. Roast nori on both sides over the flame on the kitchen stove, crush the sheets in your hands until it is almost like a powder. Soak the sweet brown rice in the water overnight. Cook the rice under a flame a little higher than medium; it will take about 30 minutes to come up to pressure. The top on the pressure cooker will not jiggle a lot. Cook for 20 minutes on a low flame. Let the pressure come down, take off the cover, and pound with a wooden pestle until half of the grains have been mashed. Wet your hands and form 2" long rectangles from the rice. These are covered with the sesame seeds, nori, and azuki beans, so that you will have red, white, and black ohagi. For the azuki bean covering, the ohagi should be a little smaller because this is a thicker covering.

Food	Amount	Protein	Methionine/Cystine gm.
Sweet brown rice	3 cups	44.4	1.41
Azuki beans		Not available	Not available
Whole sesame seeds	½ cup	38.0	2.20
Nori	3 sheets	9.6	0.46
Tamari	1 Tbsp	1.4	0.02
Total		93.4	4.09
One serving		18.6	0.81
MDR%			74%

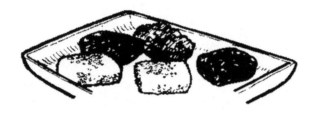

15a. Rice Salad (Serves 2)

> 1 cup cooked rice
> ½ cup onion, minced
> 1 cucumber, ¼" diced, sainome style
> ½ small cauliflower, cut into small flowerets
> 10 string beans, hasugiri style
> 5 red radishes, cut into flower shapes and kept in cold
>   water
> 3 Tbsp sesame oil
> 1½ tsp salt
> Juice of ½ lemon

Bring 1 quart of water to a boil with 1 heaping teaspoon salt. Cook the cauliflower, string beans, then carrots in this water separately until they are soft. After cooking, break the cauliflower apart, cut the string beans in ½" pieces. Heat the oil then let it cool. Add the onion and let it sit 5 minutes; add the lemon juice. Take ¼ cup of water left from cooking the vegetables and pour it over the rice to separate it into individual grains. Mix in the onion with oil; slowly mix in the carrot, string beans, cucumber, and cauliflower. Place radishes for decoration. Minced parsley can also be used for a garnish. If you wish, you can increase the quantity of rice in this recipe because there are so many vegetables.

Food	Amount	Protein	Methionine/Cystine gm.
Cooked rice	1 cup	3.7	0.11
Onion	½ cup	1.4	0.01
Cucumber	1	1.4	0.01
Cauliflower	½	2.4	Not available
String beans		Not available	Not available
Red radish	5	1.2	Not available
Sesame oil	3 Tbsp	14.3	0.83
Total		24.4	0.96
One serving		12.2	0.48
MDR%			43%

15b. Rice Salad (Serves 4)

> 4 cups cooked rice
> 2 small carrots, uncooked
> 1 small cucumber, uncooked
> ½ bunch radishes, uncooked
> ⅓ green pepper, uncooked
> 1-2 medium beets, precooked, diced, and chilled
> 4 scallions, uncooked

Dice and cut all vegetables being added to salad. Blend into chilled cooked rice by hand. If rice is glutinous, break by hand and/or rinse in cold water to make rice more flaky. Add dressing and stir thoroughly just before serving as dressing goes to the bottom while it is chilling and more salt may be needed after chilling to bring out flavors.

Dressing
   Diced raw onion
   Umeboshi juice or meat
   Dash of oil
   Dash of tamari
   Lemon juice (optional)
   Tahini (optional)

Heat oil and cool. Place diced onion and umeboshi meat in suribachi and grind together; add oil and tamari gradually to taste. Pour on top of salad and mix by hand. Place salad in refrigerator for several hours before serving. Chill thoroughly and serve immediately. This makes a delightful salad, nice for picnics. Be sure to keep it chilled until just before serving as it does turn quickly when it warms up to room temperature.

Food	Amount	Protein	Methionine/Cystine gm.
Cooked rice	4 cups	14.8	0.47
Carrot	2	2.4	0.08
Cucumber	1	0.7	0.005
Radish	½ bunch	1.2	Not available
Beets	2	0.9	0.003
Total		20.0	0.56
One serving		5.0	0.14
MDR%			13%

---

16. Tendon (Tempura With Rice And Sauce)

Sauce
   ½ cup soup stock
   1 Tbsp sake
   3 Tbsp soy sauce
   1 Tbsp mirin

Mix sauce ingredients, bring to a boil and keep hot: Dip hot tempura in sauce and decorate each bowl of hot brown rice with three pieces and pour 1 tablespoon sauce over each bowl. Cover each bowl with a rice bowl cover and serve immediately. If you use cold tempura, bring the sauce to a boil, add cold tempura, and bring to a boil without cover. Remove tempura, place on hot rice, pour 1 Tbsp of sauce over each bowl, cover each bowl, and serve.

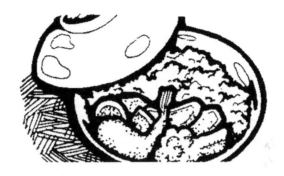

Tempura
   1 cup whole wheat pastry flour
   2 Tbsp rice flour
   1¼ cups water
   1 tsp salt
   2 tsp arrowroot starch
   1 small egg

Beat egg, salt, and water together. Mix flour into water with two thick chopsticks. Batter may be left slightly lumpy.

Heat oil. Oil should be at least 3 inches deep. Stir with chopsticks so temperature of oil is uniform. When oil is just beginning to smoke, about 330 degrees, test it to see if a drop of batter rises to the top, or if there is a "sputter" sound when a bit of salt is added. If so, oil is ready to use.

If oil is too shallow or too many pieces are dropped in at one time, temperature will fall quickly and tempura will be oily. Tempura swimming freely in oil will be crispy. Poor quality oil evaporates quickly and also gets burned (becomes dirty looking). When tempura turns light brown, turn over once and cook until both sides are the same color.

Remove tempura to upright position in a strainer set in a pan (to catch excess oil). Remove tempura from strainer to paper towels or brown paper before next batch is ready to drain.

Food	Amount	Protein	Methionine/Cystine gm.
Whole wheat flour	1 cup	16.0	0.59
Rice flour	1 Tbsp	1.9	0.06
Egg	1	6.4	0.35
Total		24.3	1.00
One serving		4.9	0.20
MDR%			18%

The following foods can be used to make tempura: prawns, shrimp, abalone, squid, broccoli, parsley, green asparagus, nori seaweed, carrots, burdock, onions, cauliflower, eggplant, sweet potatoes, green peppers, celery, shiso, and celery leaves.

For shrimp or prawns: Remove skin; leave tail on. Slice across ends of tail and squeeze out water. Slit back of prawns and remove intestines. Make 3 short cuts in short side of prawns to straighten it out and dip into batter, holding onto tail.

Abalone: Pound gently and cut into slices ¼ inch thick, 3 inches wide.

Squid: Remove skin and cut into 1½" x 3½" pieces.

Broccoli: Use flowers 3 inches long.

Parsley: Hold 2 sprigs of parsley together at bloom end, dip into batter, covering stems and half of bloom.

Asparagus: Cut into pieces 3½ inches long from tip to usable end.

Nori: Cut in half lengthwise and then into 5 strips widthwise. Holding 2 strips together, dip halfway in batter.

Carrots: Cut into ¼ inch rounds on the diagonal.

Burdock: Cut on diagonal 3 inches long, ¼ inch thick. Precook in water seasoned with tamari, if desired.

Onions: Slice into rounds ¼ inch thick.

Cauliflower: Cut as for broccoli.

Eggplant: Slice into pieces ¼ inch thick.

Sweet potatoes: Peel and cut into ½ inch strips, steam; cook until firm but not tender. Cool. Roll in pastry flour, then dip into batter.

Potatoes: Cut as for french fries.

Butternut squash: Cut into strips 1 x 3½ x ¼ inch.

Green peppers: Slice in rounds ¼ inch thick; de-seed.

Celery: Cut into 3 inch lengths.

Carrot greens: Use leafy section 5 inches long, dip only one side into batter.

Shiso leaves: Same as carrot leaves. Same for celery.

Grated ginger (for fish) and grated daikon are usually served with tempura. Daikon aids in digesting oily foods. Equal amounts of grated carrots and daikon mixed together pleases children—it is milder and colorful.

---

17. Oyster Rice—Pressure Cooked (Serves 7)

> 5 cups brown rice
> 2 Tbsp soy sauce
> ½ lb small oysters
> 7 cups water
> 1 tsp salt

Place the oysters in a strainer, sprinkle with salt, mix up well, and wash under running water. Set aside. Put the washed rice in the pressure cooker, add 1 tsp salt, cover with a regular pan cover, and bring to a boil over a hot flame for 20 minutes. Then add the oysters and soy sauce and mix slowly from top to bottom. Now lock the pressure cover on the pot and bring up to a full pressure over a high flame. When at full pressure, turn heat to low flame and cook for 45 minutes. After pressure returns to normal, serve immediately.

Food	Amount	Protein	Methionine/Cystine gm.
Brown rice	5 cups	74.0	2.35
Soy sauce	2 Tbsp	2.8	0.04
Oysters	½ lb	41.2	1.76
Total		118.0	4.15
One serving		16.8	0.59
MDR%			53%

Calculated by the values of fish in the chart given by "Amino Acid Content of Foods."

18. Shrimp-Sake Ice—Pressure Cooked (Serves 8)

> 4 cups brown rice
> ½ lb shrimp
> 5 cups water
> 1½ tsp salt
> 4 Tbsp sake

De-vein the shrimp (remove black strip from along backbone with bamboo skewer) and wash in cold water. Bring to boil 5 cups water, add shrimp, and bring to boil again over high flame. Cook until shrimp turn a red color, remove from heat, and set aside to cool.

After completely cold, take the shrimp out of the water and re-move shells. Place shrimp on a dish. Filter cooking water through cotton cloth.

After washing the rice, put it in a pressure cooker, add the shrimp water and plain water to make 5 cups altogether. Add sake and salt and bring up to a boil over a low flame for 20 minutes, then turn up high. Cook in the same way as oyster rice. Mix shrimp with hot rice and serve.

Food	Amount	Protein	Methionine/Cystine gm.
Brown rice	4 cups	59.2	1.88
Shrimp	½ lb	42.4	2.81
Total		101.6	4.69
One serving		12.7	0.58
MDR%			53%

19. Fish Rice—Pressure cooked (Serves 5)

> 2 pieces white-meat fish (2" x 3" squares)
> 2 Tbsp mirin
> 4 cups rice
> 5 cups water
> ½ Tbsp salt
> 2 Tbsp soy sauce
> 1, 4" strip dashi kombu
> 2 bunches watercress

Sprinkle fish with ½ tsp salt. Mix mirin and soy sauce. Dip fish in mirin sauce for 30 minutes. Then roast this fish on both sides on a metal toaster or fry pan. Then break up the fish into small pieces.

After washing the rice, set the kombu in the bottom of the pressure cooker, add the washed rice, and add 5 cups water. Add the leftover mirin sauce, 1 Tbsp sake, and 1 tsp salt. Cover pot with a regular cover and cook over low flame for 20 minutes. Remove kombu, replace pressure cover and bring to pressure on high flame; then turn flame low and cook for 45 minutes. Shut flame and let sit until pressure goes down.

Pass watercress through boiling water and set aside to cool. Cut into 4" pieces. Mix watercress and fish with rice and serve.

Food	Amount	Protein	Methionine/Cystine gm.
Fish	2 pieces (oz.)	20.6	0.88
Brown rice	4 cups	59.2	1.88
Soy sauce	2 Tbsp	2.8	0.04
Watercress	2 bunches (200 gm)	3.4	0.02
Total		86.0	2.82
One serving		17.2	0.56
MDR%			51%

Ojiya (Rice Gruel)

Bring to a boil twice as much soup stock as rice, add the rice, and slowly mix. Put the cover on and bring to a boil over high flame. After boiling, cook for 45-60 minutes over a low flame without stirring. When done, serve immediately. If you wait until the ojiya cools, it will be sticky like glue; so you should serve it while it is still hot.

Creating the Best Combinations for Ojiya
    1. Chicken or fish goes best with kombu stock.
    2. Vegetables or tofu goes best with kombu stock with bonita or chuba iriko.
    3. Ojiya stock should taste a little saltier than clear broth.

How to Use Various Ingredients
    Shellfish cooked for a long time get hard; so, after ojiya comes to a boil, remove the shellfish to another bowl until the ojiya has cooked completely. Then return the shellfish to the pot.
    If you have used fish and it gives the ojiya too fishy a taste, add parsley, watercress, or scallions. Mix into pot just before turning off the flame. This gives more flavor and removes the fishy smell.

Condiments for Ojiya
    Any of the following may be used. Grated fresh ginger, washed scallions, roasted crushed nori, or minced orange rind.

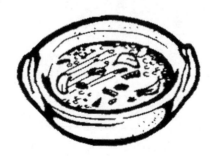

20. Shellfish Ojiya (Serves 5)

½ lb shellfish
6 cups water
6" piece dashi kombu
1 Tbsp sake (optional)
1 Tbsp soy sauce
3 cups cooked rice
1-3" carrot, sengiri style
½ lb albi, cut in quarters
1 bunch watercress

Set shellfish in a strainer into a bowl of salted water, then shake well. Bring to a boil the 6 cups water with the kombu in a heavy cast iron or stainless steel pot. Just before the water boils, remove the kombu, add the salt and tamari (and the sake if desired) and the shellfish. After it comes to a boil again, remove the shellfish. Add the cooked rice, albi, carrot and bring to a boil on high flame. Then turn low and cook for 45 minutes. Add watercress and bring to a boil again. Add the shellfish and turn off the flame. Serve immediately while it is piping hot.

Food	Amount	Protein	Methionine/Cystine gm.
Shellfish*	½ lb (227 gm)	42.5	1.81
Soy sauce	1 Tbsp	1.4	0.02
Cooked rice	3 cups	11.1	0.35
Albi	½ lb	Not available	Not available
Watercress	1 bunch (100 gm)	1.7	0.01
Total		56.7	2.19
One serving		11.3	0.44
MDR%			40%

* These values are taken from shrimp.

21. Chicken Ojiya (Serves 5)

> 6 cups water or chicken stock
> 1 Tbsp sake
> 1 bunch scallions, hasugiri style
> 1 chicken drumstick, cut into small pieces
> 1 tsp salt
> 1 Tbsp soy sauce
> 3 cups cooked rice
> ½ block tofu, cut ⅓" squares, sainome style
> 1 heaping Tbsp minced parsley

Bring chicken stock or water to boil, add sake, scallions, chicken, salt, soy sauce, and cold cooked rice. Bring to boil over high flame, then turn low and cook for 30 minutes. Add cut tofu, bring to boil, and cook 5 minutes. Shut off the flame. Sprinkle with the parsley and serve immediately.

> *Chicken Stock*
> Bones from one chicken
> 1 small onion
> 1 small carrot
> ⅓ cup chopped parsley
> 10 cups water

Break or chop chicken bones into 2-3" pieces. Add water and bring to a boil without cover. Lower flame, continue to boil and skin off scum. When stock is clear, add carrot, onion, and parsley. Continue cooking about 3 hours until about 6 cups of stock remain. Strain and use stock for cooking.

Food	Amount	Protein	Methionine/Cystine gm.
Chicken	1 drumstick	11.7	0.46
Soy sauce	1 Tbsp	1.4	0.02
Cooked rice	3 cups	11.1	0.35
Tofu, ½ block	3½ oz.	6.0	0.15
Total		30.2	0.98
One serving		6.0	0.20
MDR%			18%

22. Egg Ojiya (Serves 5)

1 Tbsp oil
1 bunch scallions
4" daikon, tanzaku style
2 tsp salt
6" carrot
6 cups soup stock
3 cups cooked rice
2-4 eggs, fertile, organic

Heat up oil, sauté scallions, add daikon and carrot, and sauté. Add the soup stock and bring to boil. Then add the salt and cooked rice; bring to boil over high flame. Turn low and cook for 45 minutes. Beat eggs then pour over the ojiya. Shut off flame. Mix and serve immediately.

Any kind of soup, i.e., vegetable, etc., is okay. You choose whichever you like. Also, you can season with miso instead of tamari. All kinds of ojiya make you feel warm; so, they are good for winter or cold days.

Food	Amount	Protein	Methionine/Cystine gm.
Carrot	6" (2 oz.)	0.7	0.03
Cooked rice	3 cups	11.1	0.35
Eggs	2-4	19.2	1.05
Total		31.0	1.43
One serving		6.2	0.29
MDR%			26%

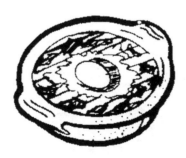

Mochi

Mochi is a special Japanese food dating from ancient times. Sweet brown rice is more Yin than regular rice and stickier. If you serve regular brown rice everyday, your stomach never grows tired. But if you eat sweet brown rice everyday, your stomach would quickly grow tired, and you would lose your appetite because it is a richer, more Yin food. So the Japanese occasionally served ohagi (sweet brown rice balls covered with sesame seeds, azuki beans, or soybean powder), mochi (pounded sweet rice), amasake (sweet rice drink), Yinnies (sweet rice candy), or mirin (sweet rice wine for cooking).

Here I would like to explain about mochi. Sweet brown rice is steamed and pounded—a yangizing process. A very condensed food, charged with mechanical energy, is produced.

All Japanese celebrate the New Year by offering a pair of round mochi, one small and large. This is displayed on the family altar to the ancestors on the kami-sama (altar to God), in the study areas, working areas, and kitchen. The round shape is smooth with no rough edges. So we hope the year ahead will go this way too, with no rough edges, but with family harmony and everything going smoothly. One Mochi is bigger than the other; the big one symbolizes the parents, the small one the offspring. Also, it represents Yin and Yang, which are never exactly identical or equal in size. Always one is greater than the other.

We decorate the top of the mochi with kombu, which stands for long life, because kombu seems to live forever, never growing old in the ocean. The Japanese say "Yoro kobu" which means "celebration of a long wonderful life." We hope the New Year will be splendid in the same way. Then a tangerine and tangerine leaves are put on top. The old word for tangerine in Japanese was "dai-dai," which means "forever." In a special prayer in which we say "dai-dai," we are expressing our hope that our children and grandchildren will continue forever and our family will never die out.

On New Year's Day, a family meal is served. Each family celebrates in their own home.

Mochi contains a very high quality starch and is very easy to digest because it is pounded and broken down. When you eat it, you get very warm and feel great vitality because the pounding compacts and compresses it. When you eat it, much energy is released. If you think this is nonsense, try it yourself.

After you eat mochi, the stomach and intestinal enzymes digest it and change it into glucose. It digests more quickly than regular rice because being more yin, the starch more easily decomposes (like fruit, which is yin and decomposes very easily).

When you eat mochi, serve it with daikon (large white radish) or natto (steamed fermented soybeans). Most people usually over-eat mochi because it is so condensed and so delicious. So, daikon and natto are served with it to help digest it.

When you eat much starch, more vitamin B1 is needed; this is found in natto and daikon.

Mochi helps people who have weak stomachs and are skinny. Sumo wrestlers eat mochi often for energy and building up their solid muscles. Japanese farmers who are very active eat mochi often to build up their bodies. In winter, Japanese country folk would save broken brown rice that is left when rice is milled. This is made into flour and added to mochi.

If a pregnant mother eats mochi often, the baby will have great durability as it grows up because the mochi gives it such a strong foundation. This foundation becomes the source of great durability later in life. Just as mochi is flexible and strong, so the child becomes like this. Mochi also helps the nursing mother produce more milk.

Mochi makes a good snack. It is especially ideal for growing children. It satisfies their desire for treats between meals and gives them a nutritious, bodybuilding food at the same time.

---

23. Mochi Making—Rice Flour Mochi (Serves 15)

> 5 cups sweet brown rice (pressure cooked)
> 7 cups sweet brown rice flour
> 5 cups water

Rinse rice in pan of water until water becomes clear. Soak 24 hours (Fig. 1). Put soaked rice in a pressure cooker, cover, and cook using a flame a little higher than medium. Bring to full pressure, turn down, and cook for 20 minutes (Fig. 2). Turn off the heat and let it stand for 45 minutes (Fig. 3). Pound with a suricogi (wooden pestle) (Fig. 4). Mix flour with very hot rice and pound again (Fig. 5). Wet both hands in cold water and knead rice (Fig. 6). Dip hands in cold water each time before handling hot rice. When most of the rice grains are broken down, the kneading process is completed.

Bring water to a boil in rice steamer. Put a wet cloth inside the pan after water begins to steam. Place mochi- flour mixture on top of the wet cloth and cover with the same cloth. Steam-cook at high heat for 20 minutes (Fig. 7). Pierce mochi with a dry chopstick—if nothing sticks to it when it is withdrawn, the mochi is done (Fig. 8). Spoon out a lump of mochi, form it into a ball, and coat it with the covering you prefer (Fig. 9). Also shape the mochi into 3" flat rounds, put a dab of cooked azuki beans in the center and fold the corners into a ball with the azuki in the center (Fig. 10). This is called daifuku.

If you have some left-over mochi, make 3" round flat balls or large loaf shapes and cover with flour. Leave this until cool then store in the freezer. This will keep for six months. When you serve it, bake or fry it first.

Food	Amount	Protein	Methionine/Cystine gm.
Sweet brown rice (cooked)	1.2 cups	17.8	0.56
Sweet brown rice flour	7 cups	103.6	3.29
Total		121.4	3.85
One serving		8.0	0.25
MDR%			21%

B. Mochi Preparation

Cut mochi the day after you have made it. You will need a cutting board, knife, and wet dishtowel. When cutting mochi, put all your weight on the knife and press down. After a while the knife will get sticky, so keep the knife wet and clean it off. If you want to store mochi dry for later use as a snack, first form the mochi into bread dough shapes and cut it into 8" thin slices or 3" square pieces

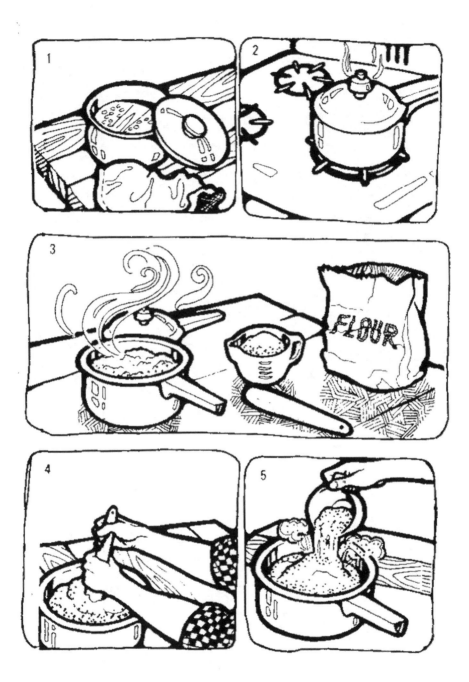

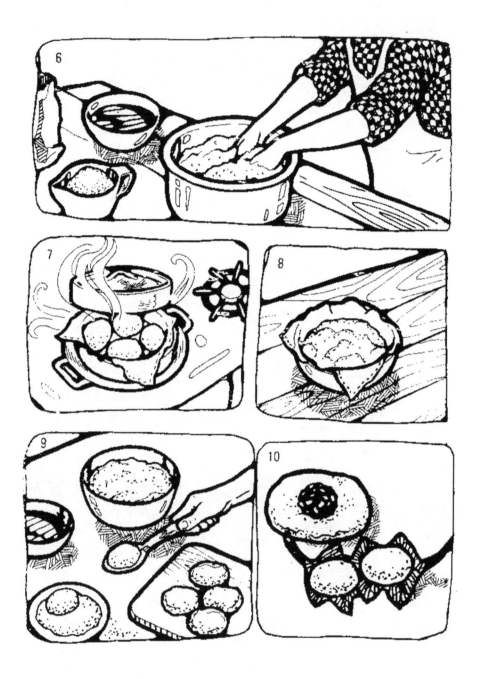

for snacks and keep in a clean dry place for 10 days. After drying, you can keep it in a covered jar for a long time. When you serve this dry mochi, toast it first in a dry fry pan or deep fry and sprinkle with salt, amasake, or Yinnie syrup. Deep fried it makes good croutons for potage, miso, or clear soup. After cutting mochi, keep it fresh in a plastic bag, tie, and freeze. It will keep a long time this way.

C. Water Mochi

If not frozen, mold will easily grow on mochi. However, this is not harmful. Just scrape it off with a knife. If it becomes very moldy and dry, scrape off the mold and soak the mochi in water. Wash off the flour and keep it covered with cold water in a cool place. Change the water after three days. After five days the mochi will get soft. Then let it drain for ½ day before using it. Cut the mochi into 1" square pieces. Heat up the iron fry pan and add mochi, cover, and toast both sides for 5 minutes with the pan covered. Repeat this toasting process until the mochi gets soft. Then you can serve it with any kind of sauce or dish.

D. Baked Mochi

To cook on top of the gas stove, a Japanese metal toaster is very useful. Turn the flame up high, put mochi on top of the metal toaster, and cover with a pie pan. This holds steam in and helps it bake more quickly. As it cooks, turn it a couple of times.

If you use the oven, preheat it to 450 degrees until the oven racks are hot (this prevents the mochi from sticking to them) and place the mochi on them to bake. If the metal rods are too widely spaced, put silver foil on top and bake the mochi for 7-10 minutes. When the mochi have puffed up, but before they pop open, take them out.

E. Deep Fried Mochi

Heat up oil to 350 degrees, shut off flame, and let sit for 5 minutes until the oil cools slightly. Add mochi, turn the flame on medium high, and fry, turning several times until both sides of the mochi become an ox-brown (medium brown). Then drain on a rack that has a reservoir for saving the oil, and transfer them to a paper towel.

When frying, don't put too many in the oil at one time because they stick together. Also, the temperature of the oil will drop too much so they won't cook well.

If the mochi tastes too oily, toast them on a metal toaster on top of the stove. This evaporates excess oil and the oily taste.

F. Boiled Mochi

After baking mochi, add it to soup and cook over medium flame. Don't use a high flame to boil mochi because it will make them dissolve. Also the soup will get thick and turbid. So always boil over medium flame. Just bringing it to a boil is enough; then you can serve it immediately.

---

24. Yaki Mochi Nabe (Mochi Stew) (Serves 6)

> ½ lb white meat fish
> 12 pieces of mochi, 2" x 3"
> 1 cup grated daikon radish
> 8 cups soup stock
> Oil for deep frying
> 2 eggs, organic, fertilized (optional)
> 1 bunch of watercress
> ½ cup flour
> *Tempura batter* (See recipe #16)
> ⅔ cup whole wheat pastry flour
> 3 Tbsp water
> 1 egg
> 2 Tbsp black sesame seeds

Deep fry mochi and drain off excess oil. Cut fish into bite size pieces, cover with flour, dip in tempura batter, and deep fry. Wash watercress and cut into 2" pieces.

Decorate a big plate with fried mochi, fish tempura, and watercress. Put grated daikon in a bowl in the center. Beat two eggs (if using) and place them in another bowl.

Bring soup stock to a boil, add 1 tsp of salt and 3 Tbsp soy sauce. Add ½ of the bowl of grated daikon to the soup stock. Add two beaten eggs and stir. Then add mochi, fish tempura, and watercress. Bring to a boil and serve immediately at the table on a small warming unit if you have one.

Keep adding more daikon, mochi, tempura, and watercress as it is used up by your guests and family.

Food	Amount	Protein	Methionine/Cystine gm.
Fish	½ lb	41.2	1.96
Mochi	12 (2" x 3")	40.0 approx.	1.28
Eggs	3	19.2	1.05
Whole wheat flour	⅔ cup	12.0	0.44
Sesame seeds	2 Tbsp	9.5	0.55
Total		121.9	5.28
One serving		20.3	0.88
MDR%			80%

---

25. Salad-Sauces for Mochi (Serves 6)

   1 tsp mustard paste
   2 Tbsp peanut butter
   ⅓ cup boiled crab
   1 piece baked or boiled salmon
   3 Chinese cabbage
   1 apple
   2 sheets nori
   2 Tbsp mayonnaise sauce
   2 Tbsp French dressing (mix 1 Tbsp rice vinegar, 2 Tbsp
      olive oil or corn oil, and ½ tsp salt)

Break salmon into small pieces and mix 1 Tbsp of mayonnaise sauce. Break crab into small pieces and mix with 1 Tbsp of french dressing.

Cut Chinese cabbage and apple into 1" long sengiri-style matchsticks. Squeeze water from cabbage and mix with French dressing.

Toast nori and cut each sheet the long way into eight pieces and put this into a serving dish. Mix the peanut butter with the mustard paste. Now, take all the salad-sauces to the table and let each person make his own choice of sauces. Finally, each one can wrap his mochi with a strip of nori and enjoy it.

Mustard paste: Make about 1 cup of strong bancha tea. Place mustard in ovenproof bowl and add 1½ Tbsp of hot tea. Stir quickly. Invert bowl over burner on low heat for about 5 minutes until mustard mixture is slightly browned and there is a potent mustard fragrance.

Food	Amount	Protein	Methionine/Cystine gm.
Peanut butter	2 Tbsp	8.4	0.22
Boiled crab	⅓ cup (2 oz.)	9.3	0.39
Boiled salmon	1	10.3	0.44
Nori	2 sheets	7.2	0.35
Total		35.2	1.40
One serving		5.9	0.23
MDR%			21%

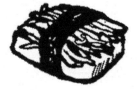 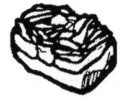

26. Bonita Mochi

Bake mochi in the oven or on top of the gas stove. Then boil it in plain water. When mochi gets soft, remove it to the serving plate. Put a drop of soy sauce on each square and top with fresh-shaved bonita. Serve immediately.

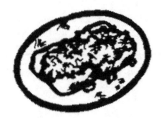

27. Orange-Miso Mochi

Mix one part barley miso (mugi) and one part rice miso (kome. Add water and a little bit of sake and mix until creamy. Bring to a boil over medium flame, stirring constantly until all water is evaporated and miso gets shiny. Set aside to cool. Mix in just enough grated orange rind to flavor it. Then spread baked mochi with this sauce and garnish with a little bit of minced orange rind.

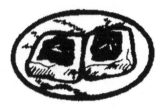

28. Oroshi Mochi—Mochi With Grated Radish

Grate daikon, squeeze out a little of the water, add a small amount of tamari, and mix. Roast nori, cut with scissors into long threadlike strips. Pass the baked mochi through boiling water. Set on serving dishes and cover each piece with grated radish. Then garnish the center with a pinch of nori strips.

29. Rolled Oats (Serves 4)

> 2 cups rolled oats
> 5 cups water
> 1 tsp salt

Roast oat flakes in a dry skillet over a medium flame until golden in color. Add 4 cups of water and salt. Return pan to stove. Bring to a boil, add remaining cup of water, and bring to a boil again, lower flame, cover, and cook until desired consistency is reached. (Adding cold water after the first boil makes a smoother cereal.) Stir occasionally during cooking. Serve with sesame salt. This cereal can be cooked the night before or slowly simmered overnight.

Food	Amount	Protein	Methionine/Cystine gm.
Rolled oats	2 cups (200 gm.)	22.8	0.84
One serving		5.7	0.21
MDR%			19%

30. Whole Oat Groats (Serves 2)

> 1 cup whole oats
> 5-6 cups water
> ½ tsp salt

After washing the groats, dry roast in a heavy skillet until golden in color, stirring constantly to prevent burning. Pour water over the oats, add salt, and bring to a boil. Cover and let simmer over a low heat for several hours or overnight.

For pressure cooking, roast the groats as above, add water and salt, and pressure cook for 1½ hours over a low flame after the pressure comes up. If made the night before, the groats can be left in cooker and reheated in the morning.

Food	Amount	Protein	Methionine/Cystine gm.
Whole oats	1 cup	11.4	0.42
One serving		5.7	0.21
MDR%			19%

31a. Bulghur (Serves 4)

Bulghur is cracked, steamed wheat, usually imported from the Near East. It tastes very light and fresh and is good for summertime. It cooks very quickly so you don't have to slave in a hot kitchen on hot summer days. And, if guests arrive suddenly, it can be prepared very quickly.

> 2 cups bulghur
> 2 cups water
> 1 Tbsp oil
> 1 tsp salt

Wash bulghur, strain, and sauté in oil for 5 minutes. Add salt and water and bring to a boil on medium flame. After boiling, cook over low flame for 15 minutes. Shut off flame. After 10 minutes, it is ready to serve.

Vegetable curry sauce is very delicious over bulghur. (See next recipe)

Food	Amount	Protein	Methionine/Cystine gm.
Bulghur	2 cups (200 gm.)	19.8	0.99
One serving		5.0	0.25
MDR%			22%

31b. Vegetable Curry Sauce (Serves 10)

> 2 onions, sliced thin
> 11 cups water
> 1 carrot, slivered
> ½ tsp curry powder
> ⅓ lb string beans, cut in 1" pieces
> 2 tsp salt
> 1 cup whole wheat pastry flour
> 3 tsp oil

Sauté onions until browned. Add carrot, curry powder, and flour. Sauté 10-15 minutes. In another pan, boil string beans in soup stock (see below) or in plain water. Add string beans and stock or water to other vegetables and flour. Boil slowly for 30 minutes. Add salt and simmer a few minutes longer.

Food	Amount	Protein	Methionine/Cystine gm.
Onion	2 (100 gm.)	1.4	0.01
Carrot	1 (50 gm.)	0.7	0.03
Whole wheat flour	1 cup	16.0	0.59
Total		18.1	0.62
One serving		1.8	0.06
MDR%			6%

31c. Kombu Stock

> Kombu, 4" x 12"
> ⅔ cup chuba iriko
> 14 cups water

Place kombu in 7 cups of water, bring to a boil with a cover. Add fish and boil again, strain, and reserve the stock. Add 7 cups more water to the stock and cook 30 minutes with cover.

---

32. Vegetable Soup with Bulghur (Serves 4)

> 2 cups bulghur
> 1 onion cut ½" pieces, mawashigiri style
> 1 stalk thyme or ¼ tsp crushed thyme
> ½ medium sized carrot cut ½" pieces, sainome style
> 1 Tbsp parsley
> 1 medium sized beet (cook whole in lightly salted water,
>   then cut ½" pieces, sainome style)
> 1 Tbsp sesame oil

Wash bulghur and strain. Add 2 cups of water, thyme, and ½ tsp salt. Bring to a boil over medium flame. Then cook for 20 minutes over low flame. Shut off heat. Heat 1 Tbsp oil. Add sliced onion and sauté until transparent. Add carrot, sauté a few minutes more, and cover with ½" water over top of vegetables. Bring to a boil, cook for 10 minutes, add 1 tsp salt, cook again for 10 minutes, add 2 tsp soy sauce, shut off, and remove from heat. Set cooked bulghur on a serving plate and cover it with vegetable soup. Decorate the center with cooked beets and sprinkle the edge with parsley. This recipe is a very colorful fresh-looking dish for summer. The bulghur is light tan, the beets deep red, and the parsley adds a rich green contrast.

Food	Amount	Protein	Methionine/Cystine gm.
Bulghur	2 cups (200 gm.)	19.8	0.99
One serving		5.0	0.25
MDR%			22%

---

33. Bulghur Croquettes

Cook bulghur and add ½ as much minced raw onion, and ¼ as much minced carrot, and 1 tsp salt. Then add whole wheat pastry flour until you can make croquettes that stick together. Shape them into round, flat, or triangular shapes, and dip in tempura batter (see recipe #16). Roll in bread crumbs, corn meal, or roasted sweet brown rice flour, and deep fry. Then set in strainer over empty pan to catch the excess oil that drips off the cooked croquettes. Use this oil in baking or sautéing. Next, place croquettes on a paper towel. Serve with grated daikon and soy sauce, which helps digest oil.

---

34. Cracked Wheat (Serves 4)

> 1 cup cracked wheat
> 1 sweet potato (cooked for 10 minutes in pressure cooker then mashed)
> 1 Tbsp oil
> 1 tsp salt
> 2 Tbsp roasted sesame seeds (black or white)

Heat up oil. Sauté cracked wheat for 5 minutes. Add 2½ cups of water and bring to a boil on medium flame. After boiling, reduce to low flame. After tender, add mashed sweet potato and 1 tsp salt, and cook 5 more minutes. Mix well, stirring constantly. Sprinkle roasted sesame seeds in bottom of casserole dish. Then add cooked cracked wheat and press down. Set aside to cool. After completely cooling, turn upside down, slice, and serve. Sesame seeds come out on top, and look very attractive. If there are yin sick people, don't use sweet potato.

Food	Amount	Protein	Methionine/Cystine gm.
Cracked wheat	1 cup (100 gm.)	13.3	0.49
Sweet potato	1 (100 gm.)	1.8	0.06
Sesame seeds	2 Tbsp	9.5	0.55
Total		24.6	1.10
One serving		6.2	0.27
MDR%			25%

---

35. Cracked Wheat with Onions (Serves 5)

> 2 cups cracked wheat
> 2 onions, chopped
> ½ tsp salt
> 3 Tbsp oil
> 6 cups boiling water

Brown wheat in frying pan with 1½ Tbsp oil until slightly colored and fragrant. Sauté onions in separate pan with the remaining oil. When onions are done, add them with salt and boiling water. Cover and let simmer for 1 hour, stirring occasionally. Add more water if necessary. (A pinch of thyme, basil, or garlic can be added to enhance flavor.)

Food	Amount	Protein	Methionine/Cystine gm.
Cracked wheat	2 cups (200 gm.)	26.6	0.98
One serving		5.3	0.196
MDR%			18%

36. Barley Kayu (Serves 2)

>1 cup pressed barley
>1 onion, minced
>5 cups water
>1 tsp salt

Wash the pressed barley, put in a saucepan, add water, and bring to a boil. Turn flame down and simmer for 4 hours or overnight. Sauté onion in 1 tsp oil and add to barley kayu. Add salt and cook for 30 minutes more. When you make barley or rice kayu, don't stir while it is cooking. After you have shut off the flame, then you can stir it.

Food	Amount	Protein	Methionine/Cystine gm.
Pressed barley	1 cup (100 gm.)	12.8	0.441
One serving		6.4	0.22
MDR%			20%

37. Corn Meal Cereal (Serves 2)

>1 cup corn meal
>¼ tsp salt
>3-4 cups boiling water
>⅛ tsp oil

Sauté corn meal in oil. Add salt and boiling water. Cook 30-35 minutes or until well done. Add tamari to taste.

Food	Amount	Protein	Tryptophan*
Corn meal	1 cup (118 gm.)	10.9	0.07
One serving		5.4	0.03
MDR%			12%

*Tryptophan is the limiting amino acid for corn.

38. Grain Milk Cereal

> 1 cup grain milk powder (kokkoh, available in stores
>   selling macrobiotic products)
> 5 cups water
> ¼ tsp salt
> ½ tsp oil

Sauté grain milk powder in oil until there is a nut-like fragrance. Cool. Add water gradually to prevent lumping. Bring to a boil on medium flame, stirring continuously from side to side to keep from sticking. (Don't use the highest flame until you get the knack of cooking cereal.) Add salt. Lower the flame and simmer until thickened. Cook about 30-45 minutes. Serve with sesame salt and/or tamari.

One cup grain milk equals the following protein amount.

Food	Amount	Protein	Methionine/Cystine gm.
Brown rice	35 gm.	7.4	0.28
+ Sweet brown rice	60 gm.		
Sesame seeds	5 gm.	2.0	0.11
Total		9.4	0.39

39. Millet (Serves 4)

> 2 cups millet
> 4 cups boiling water
> ½ tsp salt

If pressure cooking millet, roasting beforehand is not necessary. Cook just 20 minutes after pressure comes up. For boiling, add boiling water and cook 30-40 minutes with a tight cover. Serve with nitsuke vegetables or onion-tahini sauce.

Food	Amount	Protein	Methionine/Cystine gm.
Millet (pearl)	2 cups (200 gm.)	22.8	0.84
One serving		5.7	0.21
MDR%			19%

40. Millet Kayu (Serves 5)

> 1½ cups millet, washed and strained
> 6 cups water
> 1 tsp salt

Put all the ingredients in a pressure cooker, bring to pressure, and cook for 5 minutes. Remove from the stove, let it sit for 10 minutes. After 10 minutes, use cold water to bring down the remaining pressure. Serve immediately.

Food	Amount	Protein	Methionine/Cystine gm.
Millet (pearl)	1½ cups (150 gm.)	17.1	0.63
One serving		3.4	0.13
MDR%			11%

41. Buckwheat Groats (Serves 2)

> 1 cup whole buckwheat groats
> 2 cups boiling water
> ¼ tsp salt

If using white buckwheat groats, wash thoroughly and dry roast in a heavy skillet for 10 minutes or until nut brown. Or, spread groats on a cookie sheet and roast in a 350 degree oven for about 15 minutes. Already roasted groats need only to be re-roasted for 5 minutes.

Add boiling water and salt to pan and simmer over a low flame for 20 minutes. Serve with nitsuke onions or onion sauce.

Food	Amount	Protein	Methionine/Cystine gm.
Buckwheat groats	1 cup	11.5	0.42
One serving		5.7	0.21
MDR%			19%

42. Thick Buckwheat Cream (Serves 2)

> 1 cup buckwheat flour
> 2 cups boiling water
> ¼ tsp salt

Roast buckwheat flour and salt for a few minutes in a dry pan over a medium-low flame, turning the flour as needed to not burn. Add boiling water and mix vigorously. Turn off heat and serve immediately. Serve with chopped scallions and tamari.

Food	Amount	Protein	Methionine/Cystine gm.
Buckwheat flour	1 cup	11.5	0.42
One serving		5.7	0.21
MDR%			19%

43. Oat Groats with Brussels Sprouts (Serves 5)

> 2 cups oat groats
> 3 cups water
> 1 tsp salt
> 1 lb brussels sprouts
> Bread crumbs
> 2 Tbsp oil

Wash oat groats. Add water and salt and pressure cook for 1 hour. Reduce pressure. Sauté brussels sprouts in a skillet and add them to the oat groats. Place in a casserole, season with salt and/or tamari to taste. Sprinkle bread crumbs on top and place in preheated 350 degree oven and bake for 20 minutes, until the top browns evenly.

Food	Amount	Protein	Methionine/Cystine gm.
Oat groats	2 cups (160 gm.)	22.8	0.84
Brussels sprouts	1 lb	20.0	0.23
Total		42.8	1.07
One serving		8.6	0.21
MDR%			20%

44. Bulghur Gratin Casserole (Serves 4)

> 1 cup bulghur
> 1 medium onion, minced
> ½ cup whole wheat pastry flour
> 10 fresh string beans cooked in salt water and cut in thin
>   diagonal slices
> 2 tsp salt
> 2 Tbsp oil

Cook bulghur in 1 cup of water (see recipe #31a.). Mix onion, string beans, and cooked bulghur with 1 tsp salt. Set mixture in a oven-proof casserole dish. Heat 1 Tbsp oil, add flour, and sauté until a fragrant smell is given off. Set aside to cool. Then add 1½ cups of water. Mix well. Pour this batter into a casserole dish, sprinkle 1 tsp oil evenly over the top, and bake at 450 degrees until the top is lightly browned.

Food	Amount	Protein	Methionine/Cystine gm.
Bulghur	1 cup	12.4	0.62
Whole wheat flour	½ cup	8.0	0.30
Total		20.4	0.92
One serving		5.1	0.23
MDR%			21%

45. Ryeberry Casserole

> 2 cups rye berries
> 3 cups water
> ½ tsp salt

Wash rye berries. Add water and salt. Pressure cook 45 minutes. Reduce pressure to normal. Uncover and add Purple Cabbage Nitsuke (see below). Simmer together for 20-30 minutes before serving. A delicious combination that makes a nice change from ordinary combinations of grains and vegetables. For variation, crack rye berries coarsely in a Corona flour mill, wash, drain, and cook as above.

Purple Cabbage Nitsuke
  1 purple cabbage
  4 medium onions, mawashigiri style
  1-2 salt plum meats (according to taste and salt quantity
     desired)
  2 Tbsp oil

Sauté onions until clear; add cabbage that has been quartered and cut fine. Simmer until cabbage is well cooked. Season with salt plum meat.

Note: The amino acids content of rye berries is not available.

---

46. Barley-Cabbage Casserole (Serves 3)

  2 cups barley
  3 cups water
  ½ tsp salt
  1 cabbage

Wash and drain whole barley. Add water and salt and pressure cook 45 minutes. Reduce pressure, uncover, and add to this the cabbage, which has been cut and cooked nitsuke. Mix together; season with salt and tamari. Place in casserole, sprinkle bread crumbs on top, and bake in preheated 350 degree oven until golden brown.

Food	Amount	Protein	Methionine/Cystine gm.
Barley	2 cups (200 gm.)	25.6	0.88
Cabbage	1 (lb)	6.3	0.18
Total		31.9	1.06
One serving		10.6	0.35
MDR%			32%

47. Polenta Casserole (Serves 4)

> 2 cups corn meal
> 4½ cups boiling water
> ½ tsp salt

Cook corn meal in water ½ hour, stirring occasionally. Pour onto two plates, spread out, and cool until firm.

> 3 onions, sengiri style
> A handful of small mushrooms
> 2 cups water
> 1 Tbsp oil
> ¼ tsp salt
> 1 Tbsp soy sauce
> 1-2 Tbsp arrowroot flour

Sauté onion and simmer in water 20 minutes. Thicken sauce with arrowroot and season with tamari and salt. Simmer a few minutes longer. Place polenta in two layers in casserole with sauce in between and then on top. Sprinkle with mushrooms and bake in covered casserole at 350 degrees for ½ hour.

Food	Amount	Protein	Tryptophan*
Corn meal	2 cups	21.8	0.14
Soy sauce	1 Tbsp (14 gm.)	1.0	0.01
Arrowroot flour		Not available	Not available
Total		22.8	0.15
One serving		5.7	0.03
MDR%			12%

*Note: The limiting amino acid of corn meal is tryptophan.

Appendix I

Gomashio: When serving rice or other grains, you may wish to season them with goma-shio (sesame salt), which is prepared as follows: the proportion of sesame seeds to sea salt is usually about 8 to 1, but this can be varied according to your needs and taste. Roast seeds in pan on low heat, stirring constantly with a wooden spoon, until they begin to pop and can easily be crushed between your fingers. Do not burn. Roast sea salt in a separate pan (about 10 minutes for crude sea salt and 1 for white). Grind seeds and salt together in a suribachi (mortar and pestle). (A blender can be used instead but is much less effective in coating each grain of salt with oil, which helps prevent thirst.) Ready when about 80% of seeds are crushed. Keep in airtight container. Refrigerate in hot weather. Make fresh about once a week.

Tamari: A variety of soy sauce (sho-oyu), which has been naturally fermented without the use of sugar, mono-sodium-glutamate (aji-no-moto) or other unnatural chemicals, and aged for at least 18 months. It can be used sparingly at the table, but usually only in cooking.

Liquid Intake: Since cooked grains contain about 70% water, there is little need for additional liquids, particularly because most people just starting the diet have much excess liquid in their blood, cells and tissues. Also, since the kidneys, contrary to common belief, are not modern plumbing appliances (but rather complex organs whose tissues can become saturated with water, preventing normal passage and elimination of liquid) it is best to drink as little liquid as possible. But do not torture yourself. Up to about 8 ounces a day is a reasonable average for most people. Good ways to take such additional liquids, if needed and desired are: bancha tea, grain beverages (kokkoh [grain milk], rice tea, wheat tea, barley tea, etc.) or plain boiled water. (Mu tea, made from a blend of 16 herbs, is not recommended for daily use, except for specific illnesses, because it is very yang.) The amount of liquid desirable for each individual will vary considerably, depending on amount and type of activity, condition of the kidneys, climate, and other factors. (If you are living in a cold, wet climate or are relatively inactive physically, you will need less.) Let urination (3 times a day for a man, 2 for a woman are ideal) be your guide. But if you are strongly attracted to excess liquids, you are probably using too much salt or other yang foods, or too yang a preparation of foods (over-cooking, etc.)

Salt: Since Western people have a long history of meat-eating, and meat is very high in salt, we must be especially careful about the amount we use. Most of the recipes in *Zen Cookery,* for example, call for about twice as much salt as most Americans need. If in doubt, use less salt. You can always increase the amount later if you find you need more. Excess salt (and remember that goma-shio, tamari, and miso (naturally fermented, well-aged soybean paste) all contain salt—about 15%) will cause one to become very strongly drawn to yin foods (liquids, fruit, or even sugar). Whereas, a good balance of salt and liquid will make the ten-day rice diet not only very interesting and enjoyable but also most rewarding.

Chewing: Very thorough chewing (until liquid) is very important— especially for those who are just beginning to eat macrobiotically, because:

1. most of us have greatly reduced our ability to produce (transmute) from a limited diet the nutrients we need to recover and maintain our health. And the more one chews, the more food value is obtained (especially in the case of carbohydrates—most of the digestion of which occurs in the mouth—if carbohydrate digestion is not begun by the saliva, very little will occur in the stomach).

2. it is the most complete exercise for the entire body.

3. it helps to reduce over-eating.

4. it improves intuition by helping us distinguish truly nutritious foods from devitalized, unbalanced, processed foods. Through chewing we gain deeper appreciation for our foods, the environment that produced them, and those who grew and brought them to us. Without such appreciation, even though our food is good, it has much less value.

Warning: All is not painless or without difficulty as one recovers his mental and physical health through Macrobiotics. In order to cleanse the body and mind of impurities and excess, we have to release them into the bloodstream before expelling them from the body. Also, cycles of release and expulsion are irregular: large amounts of poisons are usually released during the first few days, followed by a period of previously-unimagined peace and joy, another (less difficult) period of release and expulsion, etc.

Reminder: After the initial period of all grains, or mainly all grains, gradually expand your diet, over a week or so, to the following diet, which has been planned for the average person living in an average climate (Spring in Kansas, for example): 50-70% whole grains, 20-30% cooked vegetables, 5% pressed salad and pickled vegetables, 5% beans and seaweeds, 0.5% fish, fruit, and nuts, 0-5% seasonings, and other foods, such as dairy products, spices, fowl, beer, etc. Anything you like very much may be eaten once in a great while in small quantity.

Whole Grains: Pressure-cooked, boiled, baked, in breads (preferably from flour you have milled yourself) raw, fried, etc. Rice can be served at every meal, all year round, with wheat secondarily (a delicious bread is 2 parts whole wheat flour to 1 part whole rice flour). Other grains are served less often and in smaller amounts.

Vegetables: Any locally grown that are in season. Pressed salad and pickled vegetables every meal, all year round.

Beans: Aduki, chickpeas, lentils, black beans, navy beans, kidney beans, etc. (Soybeans—boiled or in the form of natto, okara, or tofu—should be used less often as they are quite yin.)

Seaweeds: Kombu, wakame, nori, hijiki, dulse, etc.; very good for nerves: rich in minerals, including magnesium, calcium, and iodine.

Fish: Up to about twice a week, depending on the individual's age, amount and type of activity, previous eating habits, sex, climate, etc.

(For those still in the first few months or even years of Macrobiotics, it is not wise to limit animal food too severely. Our bodies have been accustomed to such foods and to limit the amount too strictly too soon will be such a strain on the body that it will eventually rebel ('binge'). The less animal food the better, but don't torture yourself. Macrobiotics is not asceticism. Red meat, however can be eliminated immediately (unless you are living at the North or South Pole), and fowl or eggs (preferably organically fed) should be used only very occasionally, if at all. (People who live in inland areas where fresh fish are not available may wish to substitute raw (unpasteurized, unhomogenized) milk or raw milk cheese for fish. But butter, cream, and yoghurt (all very yin) should be avoided.

Fruits/Nuts: It is best to eat as little fruit as possible. But desserts made from cooked nuts, currants, chestnuts, apples, etc. (pies, cookies, baked apples, etc. in cold weather—watermelon or other raw or cooked fruit in hot weather) can be eaten in small amounts without harm, in most cases. Fruit juices are extremely yin (more yin than beer) and also represent a partial food, not a whole food, and should be avoided, even in hot weather. Sugar should be eliminated as soon as possible (this includes 'raw' and brown sugar as well as white sugar). If you have difficulty avoiding sweets, reduce the intake of salt, fish, buckwheat, and other very yang foods in your diet, while increasing the amount of pressed salad and pickled vegetables. Aduki beans and/or acorn squash or butternut squash will help reduce an attraction to sweets as will plain, raw vegetables eaten in small amounts.

Seasonings: Sea salt, miso, tamari, sesame seeds, arrowroot starch, vegetable oils (mainly corn and sesame; occasionally olive oil, sunflower, safflower, and corn germ oil). Oil helps balance salt.

Other Foods: Everyone occasionally has cravings for foods he knows are not conducive to health. We recommend not too strongly resisting such urges. If one indulges in them when they first appear, enjoys them, and then returns to one's regular diet, less harm will usually result—in the long run—than if one rigidly fights the desire, which often leads to later loss of control. Such flexibility, combined with a little practical yin-yang thinking (such as organic honey is less harmful than white sugar or 1 apple is better than 3 apples) helps one stop after a more moderate amount than if one fights it all the way. Also, we can learn from bingeing: it can indicate we have been overeating (which makes imbalance and thus attraction to extremes) or that we have been eating too narrowly. Artificial chemicals (preservatives, sprays, dyes, flavoring agents, enriching materials, etc.) should be strongly avoided, although occasional use of sprayed fruits or vegetables will be okay. Any extreme (such as absolute insistence on only organic foods) leads to its opposite. Other things to avoid: foods grown in areas more than 500 miles from your home (especially to the North or South because climatic conditions to the East or West tend to be similar), and all drugs (symptomatic or 'psychedelic'—including marijuana (see *Smoking, Marijuana, and Drugs*).

In conclusion, since it has taken us many years to develop our illnesses and to greatly reduce our transmuting ability, it will also take time to redevelop this ability and to recover our physical and mental health. And the only way to do so is gradually because diet #7, or even #6 or #5, cannot be maintained for long periods of time without 'bingeing' later. Therefore, a broad, flexible diet is recommended. (See *Macrobiotics: An Invitation To Health and Happiness*, by George Ohsawa.)

It is especially important for people who have taken drugs or large amounts of sugar to eat very broadly. A reasonably strict consistent diet is the way to a life of health, happiness, and freedom. Diet #7 for a few weeks or months, followed by a few days or weeks of bingeing, #7, bingeing, etc., is not the way.

Appendix II: Protein in Rice

(From *Rice and Rice Diets* published by the Food and Agriculture Organization of the United Nations)

There is also evidence, based on rat experiments, that the proteins in polished rice are superior in biological value to the proteins of enriched wheat flour.

Experiments with rats have shown the digestibility of the proteins in both whole and milled rice to be high, namely 96.5 and 98 percent respectively.

Relatively few investigations have been done on human beings to determine the biological value and digestibility of rice proteins. The following are, however, worthy of record.

Workers in India who investigated the biological value of the proteins in an average rice eater's diet and studied the effect of replacing part of rice by other cereals, such as whole wheat flour, or wheat flour mixed with maize, millet, or barley, found that the rice proteins had a higher biological value than any of the other cereal mixtures. Similar results were obtained by Basu and his coworkers who carried out experiments with subjects on vegetarian rice and wheat diets. The digestibility coefficients were of the same order in the two sets of experiments and the value obtained for the different cereals did not differ appreciably.

Digestibility trials with four women subjects on a typical Chinese diet in which cereals or a cereal-soya meal mixture supply 60 percent of the protein intake gave the following values: rice 81.3, millet 77.8, millet-soya meal 70.6.

Appendix III:

The amounts of fat soluble vitamins A and D in rice are negligible as in other cereals. On the other hand, the Vitamin E content of whole rice is considerable. Whole rice compares well with whole wheat as a source of water-soluble vitamins, but wheat, especially high protein varieties, has a higher thiamine content. The riboflavin content of rice is low and Vitamin C is practically absent. The average thiamine, riboflavin, and niacin content of 13 varieties of brown rice (husked) has been reported to be 3.55, 0.60, and 53.08 micrograms respectively per gram.

Appendix III: Average Compositions of Rice, Wheat, and Corn

(from *Rice and Rice Diet* published by the Food and Agriculture Organization of the United Nations)

	Rice Husked	Rice Milled	Wheat Whole	Wheat White	Corn Whole
100 calorie portions (gms.)	28.0	29.0	28.0	28.0	27.0
Protein (percent)	8.9	7.6	11.1	9.3	10.0
Fat (percent)	2.0	0.3	1.7	1.0	4.3
Carbohydrate (percent)	77.2	79.4	75.5	77.2	73.4
Fuel value per 100 gm (in calories)	356.0	351.0	362.0	355.0	372.0
Ash (percent)	1.90	0.4	1.8	0.5	1.50
Fibre (percent)	1.0	0.2	2.4	0.4	2.3
Vitamins (parts per million)					
Ascorbic Acid	3-5	0.6-1.0	3.2-7.7	0.87	4.4
Thiamine	8-1.0	0.28	1-1.2	0.40	1.3-1.5
Riboflavin	55	15-20	53	10	121
Nicotinic Acid	17	6.4	13.4	5.70	8
Pantothenic Acid	10.3	4.5	4.6	2.20	
Choline Chloride					
Vitamin A (International units per gm)	5-1.0	0	0.2-0.35		7-7.5
Tocopherol			9.10	0.30	31.0
Minerals (percent)	0.084	0.009	0.50	0.020	0.015
Ca (calcium)	0.119	0.028	0.170		0.100
Mg (magnesium)	0.342	0.079	0.480		0.400
K (potassium)	0.78	0.28	0.100		0.050
Na (sodium)	0.290		0.100		

Bibliography

Macrobiotic Diet
    Macrobiotics: An Invitation To Health And Happiness by George Ohsawa, published by George Ohsawa Macrobiotic Foundation.
    Practical Guide To Far-Eastern Macrobiotic Medicine by George Ohsawa, published by George Ohsawa Macrobiotic Foundation.
    Rice and Rice Diet by Food and Agriculture Organization of the United Nations, published by the United Nations.
    Vital Facts About Foods by Otto Carque.
    Protein and Nutrition by Dr. M. Hindhede.
    Over Consumption of Protein and Under Consumption of Basic Elements by Dr. C. Roese.
    Hidden Truth of Cancer by K. Morishita, published by George Ohsawa Macrobiotic Foundation.
    Vitamin C and Fruit by George Ohsawa & Neven Henaf, published by George Ohsawa Macrobiotic Foundation.
    Zen Macrobiotics by George Ohsawa, published by George Ohsawa Macrobiotic Foundation.
    Acid and Alkaline by Herman Aihara, published by George Ohsawa Macrobiotic Foundation.
    Soybean Diet by Herman and Cornellia Aihara, published by George Ohsawa Macrobiotic Foundation.
    Smoking, Marijuana, and Drugs by George Ohsawa and Others, published by George Ohsawa Macrobiotic Foundation.

Macrobiotic Cooking:
    Chico-San Cookbook by Cornellia Aihara, published by George Ohsawa Macrobiotic Foundation.
    Do Of Cooking by Cornellia Aihara, published by George Ohsawa Macrobiotic Foundation.
    Freedom Through Cooking by Iona Teeguarden, published by Redwing Books.
    Zen Cookery by Shayne Oles, published by George Ohsawa Macrobiotic Foundation.

Art Of Just Cooking by Lima Ohsawa, published by Autumn Press.

Cooking For Life by M. Abehsera, published by Swan House.

Diet For A Small Planet by F. Lappe.

Eating For Life by N. Altman.

Macrobiotic Cooking by E. Farmilant, published by Pyramid Books.

Natural Foods Sweet Tooth Cookbook by E. Farmilant, published by Doubleday & Co., New York.

The Sweet Life by M. Newman.

Zen Macrobiotic Cooking by M. Abehsera, published by Avon.

Macrobiotic Philosophy:

Unique Principle by George Ohsawa, published by George Ohsawa Macrobiotic Foundation.

Book Of Judgement by George Ohsawa, published by George Ohsawa Macrobiotic Foundation.

Other Books from the
George Ohsawa Macrobiotic Foundation

Acid Alkaline Companion - Carl Ferré; 2009; 121 pp.

Acid and Alkaline - Herman Aihara; 1986; 121 pp.

Basic Macrobiotic Cooking, 20th Anniversary Edition - Julia Ferré; 2007; 275 pp.

Book of Judo - George Ohsawa; 1990; 150 pp.

Cancer and the Philosophy of the Far East - George Ohsawa; 1981; 165 pp.

Essential Guide to Macrobiotics - Carl Ferré; 2011; 131 pp.

Essential Ohsawa - George Ohsawa, edited by Carl Ferré; 1994; 238 pp.

Food and Intuition 101 Volume 1: Awakening Intuition - Julia Ferré; 2012; 225 pp.

Food and Intuition 101 Volume 2: Developing Intuition - Julia Ferré; 2013; 243 pp.

French Meadows Cookbook - Julia Ferré; 2008; 275 pp.

Macrobiotics: An Invitation to Health and Happiness - George Ohsawa; 1971; 128 pp.

Philosophy of Oriental Medicine - George Ohsawa; 1991; 153 pp.

Practical Guide to Far Eastern Macrobiotic Medicine - George Ohsawa; 2010; 279 pp.

Zen Cookery - G.O.M.F.; 1985; 140 pp.

Zen Macrobiotics, Unabridged Edition - George Ohsawa, edited by Carl Ferré; 1995; 206 pp.

A wide selection of macrobiotic books is available from the George Ohsawa Macrobiotic Foundation, P.O. Box 3998, Chico, CA 95965; 530-566-9765. Order toll free: 800-232-2372. Or, you may visit *www.OhsawaMacrobiotics.com* for all books and PDF downloads of many books.